Drug Interactions Guide Book

Richard Harkness, Pharm., FASCP

"This well-organized-and-written text is highly recommended for all health care consumers who desire to take an active role in the understanding and responsible usage of their medications. Health care practitioners may find this a valuable resource to recommend to patients and complement their personal library of drug information standard texts."

James W. Cooper, Ph.D., F.A.S.C.P.
Professor and Head
Department of Pharmacy Practice
University of Georgia

PRENTICE HALL
Englewood Cliffs, New Jersey 07632

Prentice-Hall International (UK) Limited, *London*
Prentice-Hall of Australia Pty. Limited, *Sydney*
Prentice-Hall Canada Inc., *Toronto*
Prentice-Hall Hispanoamericana, S.A., *Mexico*
Prentice-Hall of India Private Limited, *New Delhi*
Prentice-Hall of Japan, Inc., *Tokyo*
Simon & Schuster Asia Pte. Ltd., *Singapore*
Editora Prentice-Hall do Brasil, Ltda., *Rio de Janeiro*

© 1991 *by*

Richard Harkness

10 9 8 7 6 5 4 3 2

Library of Congress Cataloging-in-Publication Data

Harkness, Richard.
  Drug interactions guide book / Richard Harkness.
    p. cm.
  Includes index.
  ISBN 0-13-219601-8—0-13-219619-0 (pbk)
  1. Drug interactions—Handbooks, manuals, etc. I. Title.
  [DNLM: 1. Drug Interactions—handbooks. 2. Drug Therapy—adverse
effects—handbooks. QV 39 H282da]
  RM302.H366 1991
  615'.7045—dc20
  DNLM/DLC   91-3801
  for Library of Congress   CIP

ISBN 0-13-219601-8

ISBN 0-13-219619-0 (pbk)

PRENTICE HALL
Business Information Publishing Division
Englewood Cliffs, NJ 07632

Simon & Schuster, A Paramount Communications Company

Printed in the United States of America

About the Author

RICHARD HARKNESS is a consultant pharmacist who has written articles for numerous national publications, including *Pharmacy Times*, *Drug Topics*, and the *Physicians' Desk Reference for Nonprescription Drugs*. For three years, he wrote a monthly commentary column for *Drug Topics* magazine.

His published books include *OTC Handbook: What to Recommend & Why* and *Drug Interactions Handbook*, which was a forerunner of this book.

His professional memberships include the American Society of Consultant Pharmacists, American Pharmaceutical Association, Mississippi Society of Consultant Pharmacists, and Mississippi Pharmacists Association.

In 1987, he successfully completed the specialized curriculum of *Pharmacy Practice for the Geriatric Patient*, and he has a practice specializing in consulting to long-term care facilities.

He currently writes a weekly newspaper column on consumer medical topics called *Pills & Ills*.

PROFESSIONAL DRUG INTERACTIONS SOURCES

Professionals who need more detailed information on drug interactions may consult one of the many professional references, including:

Drug Interactions Facts

Facts and Comparisons Division
J.B. Lippincott Co.
111 West Port Plaza, Suite 423
St. Louis, Missouri 63146–3098
314 878–2515

Hansten's Drug Interactions

Lea & Febiger, publisher
Applied Therapeutics, Inc.
POB 5077
Vancouver, WA 98668–5077
206 253–7123

Evaluations of Drug Interactions

American Pharmaceutical Association
2215 Constitution Avenue, NW
Washington, DC 20037
202 628–4410

Contents

Introduction

Drug interactions pose a very real problem to thousands of people each year. Often, busy physicians and pharmacists do not have the time to closely monitor for the adverse effects of drug interactions in every patient. Many patients receive multiple drug therapy—including nonprescription medications they may take on their own—and their situations warrant even greater concern. Several studies have evaluated the frequency of occurrence of drug interactions. In a study[1] of typical patients in a community medical practice, 9.2% were prescribed drugs known to interact. Of these potential interactions, 72% were considered of "moderate" clinical significance and 17% were of "major" significance. A study[2] of hospitalized patients found at least one clinically significant drug interaction in 17% of patients. Another study[3] of patients aged 60 years or over found that 32% were taking five or more drugs concurrently. Potential interactions were categorized as highly significant for 27% of the drug-drug combinations, and for 11% of the drug-alcohol and 3% of the drug-food combinations. People are recognizing more and more the need to become active partners in their own health care. Drug interactions is an area in which everyone—patient, physician, pharmacist, nurse—can work together for the benefit of the patient.

In my practice as a consultant pharmacist to long-term care facilities such as nursing homes, I notify the prescribing physician when I identify a potential drug interaction. Often, the physician had been blaming a patient's adverse symptoms or lack of proper response to a medication on some unknown cause or on the disease/illness being treated. With the realization that a drug interaction is the most likely cause, the physician can adjust the doses or times of administration of medications to alleviate the problem.

The purpose of this book is to provide a reliable, easy-to-use reference guide on adverse drug interactions and what to do about them. It is written for the layperson, yet its comprehensiveness makes it suitable for medical practitioners as well. The focus is on *clinically significant* drug interactions, so you don't have to waste your time

1. Dambro MR et al. Drug interactions in a clinic using COSTAR. Comput Biol Med. 1988. 18(1). P 31-8.

2. Durrence CW et al. Potential drug interactions in surgical patients. Am J Hosp Pharm. 1985 Jul. 42(7). P 1553-6

3. Kurfees JF et al. Drug interactions in the elderly. J Fam Pract. 1987 Nov. 25(5). P 477-88.

poring over scores of interactions that rarely occur, or may occur only theoretically. (A few exceptions are made for interactions which, though they don't have the strongest documentation, involve agents the average person is likely to encounter routinely, for example, certain vitamins.)

QUESTIONS AND ANSWERS ABOUT DRUG INTERACTIONS

What is a drug interaction?

Simply stated, a drug interaction occurs whenever one drug alters the effect of another drug. The drug altered may be made less active or more active.

What happens if you take interacting drugs?

There may be variations in individual reactions. Influencing factors include your genetic makeup, kidney and liver function, age, whether you have underlying illnesses or diseases, the amount of the drugs taken, the duration of therapy, the time interval between taking the drugs, and which drug is taken first.

Some interactions can have acutely dangerous effects. More common are interactions that cause an increase in adverse side effects or a decrease in therapeutic effect of a medication with the result that the patient doesn't feel as well as he should or doesn't get well as quickly as he should. Or chronic diseases such as high blood pressure, diabetes, and heart disease may not be controlled properly. If the physician is unaware of a drug interaction, he might make faulty treatment decisions, compounding the potential for harm.

How exactly do drugs interact?

As background, here is a simplified pharmacology lesson: A drug taken by mouth goes through four basic processes in the body. It passes into the stomach and intestinal tract. From there it is *absorbed* into the bloodstream and *distributed* throughout the body where it exerts its effects. It is then broken down or *metabolized* by the liver. Finally, this broken-down form is *excreted* (eliminated from the body) by the kidneys in the urine.

In a drug interaction, one drug modifies one or more of these processes on the other drug. This type of interaction is called a *pharmacokinetic* interaction.

The other primary type of interaction is called a *pharmacologic* interaction, with the most common being an "add on" (synergistic) interaction in which drugs with similar effects add together to increase the common effect significantly beyond that of either drug alone. The other form of this type of interaction is a "subtract from" (antagonistic) interaction, in which each drug decreases the effect of the other drug.

Does this mean that interacting drugs cannot be taken together?

Not necessarily. Usually, the dose or time of administration of one drug can be altered to offset adverse effects. Some interactions are beneficial and are deliberately exploited for this reason. There are many cases, however, in which certain drugs should not be taken together under any circumstances. The important thing is for the physician to be made *aware* of a potential interaction so that knowledgeable action can be taken to prevent harm.

SPECIAL FEATURES OF THIS BOOK

Among the special features included in this book are:

- Interactions relating to cigarette smoking, food, and vitamins.
- Graphics: easy-to-grasp circles rate severity and probability of interactions, and arrows show whether a drug's effect is increased or decreased by the interaction.
- Information on medical conditions the interacting drugs are used to treat.
- Listing of adverse symptoms (resulting from the interaction) to watch for.
- Comprehensive text listings of individual interacting drugs by both generic and brand names.

- Easy-to-use index:

  —Comprehensive listings ensure you don't overlook an inter-action—for example, looking up "cigarette" or "cigar" or "pipe" or "tobacco" refers you to "smoking" interactions listings.

  —Shows generic name and brand name side-by-side.

  —Listing of drugs by either generic or brand name sends you directly to the primary interaction index listing.

- For ease in distinguishing between brand and generic names, brand names are capitalized and generic names are not.

- "Add-on" interactions are presented as a separate supplement to the regular interactions listings, since they are so common and can be among the most dangerous.

- Special section on diseases/disorders and the drugs used to treat them.

- Special section on food-drug interactions.

- For the professional, the *Drug Interactions Guide Book* is a quick, dependable first reference source that may be the only reference a busy professional needs.

How to Use
Drug Interactions
Guide Book

Use the index to look up a drug by either its brand name or generic name. (Note that brand names are capitalized and generic names are not.) The interactions listings are shown for that drug. Sometimes you are referred to a drug "family" name. If so, go to that name in the index to see the interactions listings involving the drug in question.

Index listings refer you to an *interactions number*, not a page number, in the text. These numbers are in sequential order in the text. Look up the number to find detailed information concerning the interaction.

Example: Looking up *Valium* or its generic name, *diazepam,* shows:

Valium (diazepam) (see   diazepam (Valium) (see
     benzodiazepines)   benzodiazepines)

Looking up *benzodiazepines* (the drug "family" name) shows:

alcohol (ethanol) 7
aminophylline (Somophyllin) 36
beer 7
birth control pills 31

Turn to interaction number 31 in the text for a discussion of the interaction between Valium (diazepam) and birth control pills. Individual benzodiazepine drugs that may interact are listed by both generic and brand name in the column beneath "benzodiazepines" in the text listing.

In the text, each interaction listing shows:

*Individual interacting drugs by generic and brand names.

*SEVERITY (how potentially hazardous the interaction is).

*PROBABILITY (how likely the interaction is to occur).

*USES (medical conditions the interacting drugs are used for).

*EFFECT (states which drug's effect is increased or decreased).

*RESULT (potential consequences and adverse symptoms to watch for).

*WHAT TO DO (action to take to prevent or minimize the interaction).

SEVERITY and PROBABILITY are shown graphically with a three-circle rating. Examples:

Severity: ●●●
Probability: ●○○

One filled circle indicates *least* on the three-circle scale, two filled circles *moderate*, and three filled circles *most*. Remember that the interactions in this book are clinically significant, so that even one circle (least) has meaning.

An up or down graphic arrow beside a particular drug (usually the first drug listed) indicates whether the drug's effect is increased or decreased by the interaction. For example:

49.   ↓ birth control pills   penicillins

See the separate section on ADD-ON DRUG INTERACTIONS for information on the dangers of taking stimulant or depressant drugs together. FOOD-DRUG INTERACTIONS are presented as a special appendix.

The section on DISEASES/DISORDERS and the drugs used to treat them is included as extra information.

The interactions in this book were compiled from and cross-checked among primary and secondary source materials.

CAUTION:

THE "WHAT TO DO" SECTION IN EACH INTERACTION LISTING IS INCLUDED TO PROVIDE GUIDANCE TO THE MEDICAL PRACTITIONER AND AS INFORMATION FOR THE USER. DO NOT TRY TO MANAGE AN INTERACTION ON YOUR OWN UNLESS THE "WHAT TO DO" INVOLVES SOMETHING SIMPLE SUCH AS TAKING THE INTERACTING DRUGS 1-2 HOURS APART. HANDLING MOST INTERACTIONS REQUIRES THE EXPERTISE OF YOUR MEDICAL PRACTITIONER, WHO MIGHT NEED TO MONITOR DRUG BLOOD LEVELS, ADJUST DOSES, AND HAVE YOU REPORT ADVERSE SYMPTOMS. NEVER ADJUST DRUG DOSES OR STOP TAKING A PRESCRIBED DRUG ON YOUR OWN.

Add-on Drug Interactions: Depressants and Stimulants

Synergistic or "add-on" interactions can occur when depressant drugs are taken together or when stimulant drugs are taken together. "Add-on" means that the effects of two drugs add together to increase the primary effect significantly beyond that of either drug alone.

Add-on interactions are potentially the most common type since drugs causing depressant or stimulant effects are widely used and many are available as nonprescription products. Moreover, add-on interactions can be among the most dangerous.

ADD-ON DRUG INTERACTIONS: DEPRESSANTS

Several classes of drugs have a depressant effect. When two or more drugs from any of these classes are taken together, "add-on" or excessive physical depression and impairment can occur.

RESULT: Excessive central nervous system depression with drowsiness, dizziness, loss of muscle coordination and alertness; in severe cases, failure of blood circulation and breathing functions causing coma and death.

Listed below are depressant drug classes and lists of individual drugs in each. For ease in reference, drug lists are presented in alphabetical order two ways: by generic name and by brand name.

Be aware of potentially dangerous add-on depressant drug interactions when you take drugs from any of the following classes:

DEPRESSANT DRUG CLASSES

Alcohol
Antianxiety agents/tranquilizers
Anticholinergics
Anticonvulsants
Antidepressants (non-MAO Inhibitor type)
Antihistamines
Antipsychotics
Fenfluramine
High blood pressure drugs (centrally acting)
Muscle Relaxants
Narcotics
Propoxyphene
Sleep inducers

ALCOHOL (ethanol)

beer, liquor, wine, etc.

ANTIANXIETY AGENTS/TRANQUILIZERS (benzodiazepines and non-benzodiazepines)

Antianxiety agents are used for anxiety disorders and for the short-term relief of the symptoms of anxiety.

Antianxiety Agents/Tranquilizers (benzodiazepines):

By generic name
alprazolam (Xanax)
chlordiazepoxide (Librium)
clonazepam (Klonopin)
clorazepate (Tranxene)
diazepam (Valium)
flurazepam (Dalmane)
halazepam (Paxipam)
lorazepam (Ativan)
midazolam (Versed)
oxazepam (Serax)
prazepam (Centrax)
quazepam (Doral)
temazepam (Restoril)
triazolam (Halcion)

By brand name
Ativan (lorazepam)
Centrax (prazepam)
Dalmane (flurazepam)
Doral (quazepam)
Halcion (triazolam)
Klonopin (clonazepam)
Librium (chlordiazepoxide)
Paxipam (halazepam)
Restoril (temazepam)
Serax (oxazepam)
Tranxene (clorazepate)
Valium (diazepam)
Versed (midazolam)
Xanax (alprazolam)

Antianxiety Agents/Tranquilizers (non-benzodiazepines):

By generic name
buspirone (BuSpar)
  (Note: may not interact)
chlormezanone (Trancopal)
doxepin (Adapin, Sinequan)
droperidol (Inapsine)
hydroxyzine (Atarax,
  Vistaril)
meprobamate

By brand name
Adapin (doxepin)
Atarax (hydroxyzine)
BuSpar (buspirone)
  (Note: may not interact)
Deprol (meprobamate)
Equagesic (meprobamate)
Equanil (meprobamate)
Inapsine (droperidol)

Deprol, Equagesic, Equanil,   Meprospan (meprobamate)
Meprospan, Miltown, PMB   Miltown (meprobamate)
                                  PMB (meprobamate)
                                  Sinequan (doxepin)
                                  Trancopal (chlormezanone)
                                  Vistaril (hydroxyzine)

ANTICHOLINERGICS

Anticholinergics are used primarily for stomach and digestive tract disorders and to control tremors resulting from Parkinson's disease or from treatment with antipsychotic drugs.

By generic name   *By brand name*
atropine   Akineton (biperiden)
atropine/scopolamine/   Anaspaz (hyoscyamine)
  hyoscyamine   Artane (trihexyphenidyl)
    Barbidonna, Donnatal   Banthine (methantheline)
    Kinesed   Barbidonna
belladonna   atropine/scopolamine/
benztropine (Cogentin)   Bentyl (dicyclomine)
biperiden (Akineton)   Cogentin (benztropine)
clidinium (Quarzan)   Disipal (orphenadrine)
dicyclomine (Bentyl)   Ditropan (oxybutynin)
glycopyrrolate (Robinul)   atropine/scopolamine/
hyoscyamine (Anaspaz)   Kemadrin (procyclidine)
methantheline (Banthine)   Kinesed
orphenadrine (Disipal)   atropine/scopolamine/
oxybutynin (Ditropan)   Pathilon (tridihexethyl)
procyclidine (Kemadrin)   Pro-Banthine (propantheline)
propantheline (Pro-Banthine)   Quarzan (clidinium)
scopolamine   Robinul (glycopyrrolate)
  Transderm Scop   Transderm Scop (scopolamine)
tridihexethyl (Pathilon)
trihexyphenidyl (Artane)

ANTICONVULSANTS

Anticonvulsants are used for seizure disorders such as epilepsy.

By generic name
carbamazepine
  Epitol, Tegretol
clonazepam (Klonopin)
clorazepate (Tranxene)
diazepam
  Valium, Valrelease
ethosuximide (Zarontin)
ethotoin (Peganone)
magnesium sulfate
mephenytoin (Mesantoin)
methsuximide (Celontin)
paramethadione (Paradione)
phenacemide (Phenurone)
phenobarbital
phensuximide (Milontin)
phenytoin (Dilantin)
primidone (Mysoline)
trimethadione (Tridione)
valproic acid (Depakene)

By brand name
Celontin (methsuximide)
Depakene (valproic acid)
Dilantin (phenytoin)
Epitol (carbamazepine)
Klonopin (clonazepam)
Mesantoin (mephenytoin)
Milontin (phensuximide)
Mysoline (primidone)
Paradione (paramethadione)
Peganone (ethotoin)
Phenurone (phenacemide)
Tegretol (carbamazepine)
Tranxene (clorazepate)
Tridione (trimethadione)
Valium (diazepam)
Valrelease (diazepam)
Zarontin (ethosuximide)

ANTIDEPRESSANTS (non-MAO Inhibitor type)

Antidepressants are used for clinical depression.

By generic name
amitriptyline (Elavil, Endep)
amoxapine (Asendin)
clomipramine (Anafranil)
desipramine
  Norpramin, Pertofrane
doxepine (Adapin, Sinequan)
imipramine (Tofranil)
maprotiline (Ludiomil)
nortriptyline (Aventyl,
  Pamelor)
protriptyline (Vivactil)

By brand name
Adapin (doxepine)
Anafranil (clomipramine)
Asendin (amoxapine)
Aventyl (nortriptyline)
Desyrel (trazodone)
Elavil (amitriptyline)
Endep (amitriptyline)
Ludiomil (maprotiline)
Norpramin (desipramine)
Pamelor (nortriptyline)
Pertofrane (desipramine)

trazodone (Desyrel)　　　　　　　Sinequan (doxepine)
trimipramine (Surmontil)　　　　　Surmontil (trimipramine)
　　　　　　　　　　　　　　　　Tofranil (imipramine)
　　　　　　　　　　　　　　　　Vivactil (protriptyline)

ANTIHISTAMINES

Antihistamines are used to relieve the symptoms of allergies. (Check labels on multi-ingredient cold/cough/allergy products—many contain antihistamines.)

By generic name
astemizole (Hismanal)
azatadine (Optimine)
brompheniramine (Dimetane)
carbinoxamine (Clistin)
chlorpheniramine
　Chlor-Trimeton
clemastine (Tavist)
cyproheptadine (Periactin)
dexchlorpheniramine
　Polaramine
diphenylpyraline (Hispril)
diphenhydramine (Benadryl)
methdilazine (Tacaryl)
phenindamine (Nolahist)
promethazine (Phenergan)
pyrilamine (Nisaval)
terfenadine (Seldane)
trimeprazine (Temaril)
tripelennamine (PBZ)
triprolidine (Actidil)

By brand name
Actidil (triprolidine)
Benadryl (diphenhydramine)
Chlor-Trimeton
　chlorpheniramine
Clistin (carbinoxamine)
Dimetane (brompheniramine)
Hismanal (astemizole)
Hispril (diphenylpyraline)
Nisaval (pyrilamine)
Nolahist (phenindamine)
Optimine (azatadine)
PBZ (tripelennamine)
Periactin (cyproheptadine)
Phenergan (promethazine)
Polaramine
　dexchlorpheniramine
Seldane (terfenadine)
Tacaryl (methdilazine)
Tavist (clemastine)
Temaril (trimeprazine)

ANTIPSYCHOTICS

Antipsychotics are used for brain disorders such as schizophrenia, paranoia, and manic-depressive illness.

By generic name
acetophenazine (Tindal)
chlorpromazine (Promapar,
　Thorazine)
chlorprothixene (Taractan)

By brand name
Cibalith-S (lithium)
Clozaril (clozapine)
Compazine
　prochlorperazine

clozapine (Clozaril)
fluphenazine (Permitil,
   Prolixin)
haloperidol (Haldol)
lithium
   Eskalith, Lithane, Lithotabs,
   Lithobid, Cibalith-S
loxapine (Loxitane)
mesoridazine (Serentil)
molindone (Moban)
perphenazine (Trilafon)
pimozide (Orap)
prochlorperazine
   Compazine
promazine (Sparine)
thioridazine (Mellaril)
thiothixene (Navane)
trifluoperazine (Stelazine)
triflupromazine (Vesprin)

Eskalith (lithium)
Haldol (haloperidol)
Lithane (lithium)
Lithobid (lithium)
Lithotabs (lithium)
Loxitane (loxapine)
Mellaril (thioridazine)
Moban (molindone)
Navane (thiothixene)
Orap (pimozide)
Permitil (fluphenazine)
Promapar (chlorpromazine)
Serentil (mesoridazine)
Sparine (promazine)
Stelazine (trifluoperazine)
Taractan (chlorprothixene)
Thorazine (chlorpromazine)
Tindal (acetophenazine)
Trilafon (perphenazine)
Vesprin (see triflupromazine)

FENFLURAMINE (Pondimin)

Fenfluramine is an appetite suppressant.

HIGH BLOOD PRESSURE DRUGS (centrally-acting)

High blood pressure drugs are used to lower the blood pressure.

By generic name
clonidine (Catapres,
   Combipres)
guanabenz (Wytensin)
methyldopa
   Aldoclor, Aldomet
   Aldoril
reserpine-type
   deserpidine (Enduronyl,
      Harmonyl, Oreticyl)
   rauwolfia (Raudixin, Rauzide)

By brand name
Aldoclor (methyldopa)
Aldomet (methyldopa)
Aldoril (methyldopa)
Catapres (clonidine)
Combipres (clonidine)
Demi-Regroton (reserpine)
Demi-Salutensin (reserpine)
Diupres (reserpine)
Diutensin-R (reserpine)
Enduronyl (deserpidine)

reserpine
  Demi-Regroton,
  Demi-Salutensin, Diupres,
  Diutensen-R, H-H-R
  Hydromox R, Hydropres
  Regroton, Renese-R,
  Salutensin, Ser-Ap-Es,
  Serpasil,
  Serpasil-Apresoline,
  Serpasil-Esidrix

H-H-R (reserpine)
Harmonyl (deserpidine)
Hydromox R (reserpine)
Hydropres (reserpine)
Oreticyl (deserpidine)
Raudixin (rauwolfia)
Rauzide (rauwolfia)
Regroton, (reserpine)
Renese-R (reserpine)
Salutensin (reserpine)
Ser-Ap-Es (reserpine)
Serpasil (reserpine)
Serpasil-Apresoline
  reserpine
Serpasil-Esidrix (reserpine)
Wytensin (guanabenz)

MUSCLE RELAXANTS

Muscle relaxants are used to relieve the discomfort associated with acute, painful musculoskeletal conditions.

By generic name
baclofen (Lioresal)
carisoprodol (Rela, Soma)
chlorphenesin (Maolate)
chlorzoxazone
  Paraflex, Parafon Forte DSC
cyclobenzaprine (Flexeril)
dantrolene (Dantrium)
diazepam (Valium,
  Valrelease)
metaxalone (Skelaxin)
methocarbamol (Robaxin,
  Robaxisal)
orphenadrine (Norflex,
  Norgesic)

By brand name
Dantrium (dantrolene)
Flexeril (cyclobenzaprine)
Lioresal (baclofen)
Maolate (chlorphenesin)
Norflex (orphenadrine)
Norgesic (orphenadrine)
Paraflex (chlorzoxazone)
Parafon Forte DSC
  chlorzoxazone
Rela (carisoprodol)
Robaxin (methocarbamol)
Robaxisal (methocarbamol)
Skelaxin (metaxalone)
Soma (carisoprodol)
Valium (diazepam)
Valrelease (diazepam)

NARCOTICS

Narcotics are used for pain. Some may be used for cough or diarrhea.

By generic name
alfentanil (Alfenta)
buprenorphine (Buprenex)
butorphanol (Stadol)
codeine
   Empirin w/Codeine
   Esgic w/Codeine
   Fiorinal w/Codeine
   Phenaphen w/Codeine
   Tylenol w/Codeine
dihydrocodeine
   Synalgos-DC
fentanyl (Sublimaze)
hydrocodone
   Anexia, Lortab, Norcet,
   Vicodin, Zydone
hydromorphone (Dilaudid)
levorphanol
   Levo-Dromoran
meperidine
   Demerol, Mepergan,
   Mepergan Fortis
methadone (Dolophine)
morphine (MS-Contin)
nalbuphine (Nubain)
opium (Pantopon, Paregoric)
oxycodone
   Percocet, Percodan,
   Percodan-Demi, Roxicet,
   Roxicodone, Tylox
oxymorphone (Numorphan)
pentazocine (Talacen,
   Talwin)
sufentanil (Sufenta)

By brand name
Alfenta (alfentanil)
Anexia (hydrocodone)
Buprenex (buprenorphine)
Demerol (meperidine)
Dilaudid (hydromorphone)
Dolophine (methadone)
Empirin w/Codeine (codeine)
Esgic w/Codeine (codeine)
Fiorinal w/Codeine (codeine)
Levo-Dromoran (levorphanol)
Lortab (hydrocodone)
Mepergan (meperidine)
Mepergan Fortis (meperidine)
MS-Contin (morphine)
Norcet (hydrocodone)
Nubain (nalbuphine)
Numorphan (oxymorphone)
Pantopon (opium)
Paregoric (opium)
Percocet (oxycodone)
Percodan (oxycodone)
Percodan-Demi (oxycodone)
Phenaphen w/Codeine
   codeine
Roxicet (oxycodone)
Roxicodone (oxycodone)
Stadol (butorphanol)
Sublimaze (fentanyl)
Sufenta (sufentanil)
Synalgos-DC
   dihydrocodeine
Talacen (pentazocine)
Talwin (pentazocine)
Tylenol w/Codeine (codeine)
Tylox (oxycodone)
Vicodin (hydrocodone)
Zydone (hydrocodone)

PROPOXYPHENE

Propoxyphene is used for pain.

    Darvocet-N
    Darvon Compound-65
    Darvon
    Darvon-N
    Dolene
    Propacet
    Wygesic

SLEEP INDUCERS (barbiturates and non-barbiturates)

Sleep inducers are used for insomnia and for sedation.

Sleep Inducers (barbiturates):

By generic name	*By brand name*
amobarbital (Amytal)	Alurate (aprobarbital)
aprobarbital (Alurate)	Amytal (amobarbital)
butabarbital (Butisol)	Butisol (butabarbital)
butalbital	Lotusate (talbutal)
mephobarbital (Mebaral)	Mebaral (mephobarbital)
pentobarbital (Nembutal)	Mysoline (primidone)
phenobarbital	Nembutal (pentobarbital)
primidone (Mysoline)	Seconal (secobarbital)
secobarbital (Seconal)	
talbutal (Lotusate)	

Sleep Inducers (non-barbiturates):

By generic name	*By brand name*
chloral hydrate (Noctec)	Ativan (lorazepam)
diphenhydramine	Compoz (diphenhydramine)
Compoz, Dormarex 2, Nervine	Dalmane (flurazepam)
Nytol, Sleep-Eze 3	Doral (quazepam)
Sominex 2, Twilite	Doriden (glutethimide)
doxylamine (Unisom)	Dormarex 2
estazolam (ProSom)	diphenhydramine
ethchlorvynol (Placidyl)	Halcion (triazolam)

ethinamate (Valmid)
flurazepam (Dalmane)
glutethimide (Doriden)
lorazepam (Ativan)
methyprylon (Noludar)
paraldehyde (Paral)
quazepam (Doral)
temazepam (Restoril)
triazolam (Halcion)

Nervine (diphenhydramine)
Noctec (chloral hydrate)
Noludar (methyprylon)
Nytol (diphenhydramine)
Paral (paraldehyde)
Placidyl (ethchlorvynol)
Restoril (temazepam)
Sleep-Eze 3
   diphenhydramine
Sominex 2
   diphenhydramine
Twilite
   diphenhydramine
Unisom (doxylamine)
Valmid (ethinamate)

ADD-ON DRUG INTERACTIONS: STIMULANTS

Several classes of drugs have a stimulant effect. When two or more drugs from any of these classes are taken together, "add-on" or excessive physical stimulation can occur.

RESULT: Excessive central nervous system stimulation with nervousness, agitation, tremors, rapid heart beat, heart palpitations, fever, loss of muscle coordination, rapid, shallow breathing, insomnia; in severe cases, a dangerous rise in blood pressure can occur, indicated by headache, visual disturbances, or confusion.

[Note: Be aware that stimulants can *antagonize* the effects of drugs taken for high blood pressure, and that some stimulants (most likely nasal decongestants and nonprescription diet pills) can antagonize the effects of insulin and oral drugs taken for diabetes.]

Listed below are stimulant drug classes and lists of individual drugs in each. For ease in reference, drug lists are presented in alphabetical order two ways: by generic name and by brand name.

Be aware of potentially dangerous add-on stimulant drug interactions when you take drugs from any of the following classes:

STIMULANT DRUG CLASSES

Antidepressants (MAO Inhibitor type)
Appetite suppressants (amphetamines and non-amphetamines)
Asthma drugs (sympathomimetics and theophyllines)
Caffeine
Decongestants, Nasal
Methylphenidate
Pemoline

ANTIDEPRESSANTS (MAO Inhibitor type)

Antidepressants of the MAO Inhibitor (monoamine oxidase inhibitor) type are used for some cases of clinical depression.

By generic name	*By brand name*
isocarboxazid (Marplan)	Eutonyl (pargyline)
pargyline (Eutonyl)	Marplan (isocarboxazid)
phenelzine (Nardil)	Nardil (phenelzine)
tranylcypromine (Parnate)	Parnate (tranylcypromine)

APPETITE SUPPRESSANTS (amphetamines and non-amphetamines)

Appetite suppressants are used for short-term therapy in a weight loss program. [Amphetamine products also are used for narcolepsy (uncontrollable desire to sleep) and Attention Deficit Disorder with Hyperactivity in children.]

Appetite Suppressants (amphetamines):

By generic name	*By brand name*
amphetamine	Biphetamine
benzphetamine (Didrex)	dextroamphetamine
dextroamphetamine	Desoxyn (methamphetamine)
Biphetamine, Dexedrine	Dexedrine
methamphetamine (Desoxyn)	dextroamphetamine
	Didrex (benzphetamine)

Appetite Suppressants (non-amphetamines):

By generic name
(Prescription-only)
  diethylpropion (Tenuate)
  fenfluramine (Pondimin)
  mazindol (Sanorex)
  phenmetrazine (Preludin)
  phentermine (Ionamin)
(Nonprescription)
  phenylpropanolamine
   Acutrim, Appedrine, Control
   Prolamine, Unitrol
   Dex-A-Diet, Dexatrim

By brand name
(Prescription-only)
  Ionamin (phentermine)
  Pondimin (fenfluramine)
  Preludin (phenmetrazine)
  Sanorex (mazindol)
  Tenuate (diethylpropion)
(Nonprescription)
  Acutrim
   phenylpropanolamine
  Appedrine
   phenylpropanolamine
  Control
   phenylpropanolamine
  Dex-A-Diet
   phenylpropanolamine
  Dexatrim
   phenylpropanolamine
  Prolamine
   phenylpropanolamine
  Unitrol
   phenylpropanolamine

ASTHMA DRUGS (sympathomimetics and theophyllines)

Asthma drugs help open up constricted air passages to allow easier breathing.

Asthma Drugs (sympathomimetics):

By generic name
albuterol (Proventil, Ventolin)
bitolterol
  Tornalate
ephedrine
  Efed II, Ephedrine Sulfate

By brand name
Adrenalin Chloride
  epinephrine
Aerolone (isoproterenol)
Alupent (metaproterenol)
Arm-a-Med Isoproterenol
Arm-a-Med Isoetharine

epinephrine
  Adrenalin Chloride,
  AsthmaHaler, AsthmaNefrin
  Bronitin Mist, Bronkaid Mist
  Dey-Dose, Epinephrine
  Medihaler-Epi, microNefrin
  Primatene Mist, S-2 Inhalant
  Sus-Phrine, Vaponefrin
ethylnorepinephrine
  Bronkephrine
isoetharine
  Arm-a-Med Isoetharine
  Beta-2, Bronkometer
  Bronkosol, Dey-Lute
  Disorine, Dispos-a-Med
isoproterenol
  Isoetharine
  Aerolone, Arm-a-Med
  Isoproterenol, Dey-Dose
  Isoproterenol, Dispos-a-Med
  Isoproterenol, Isuprel,
  Medihaler-Iso, Vapo-Iso
metaproterenol (Alupent,
  Metaprel)
pirbuterol (Maxair)
terbutaline
  Brethaire, Brethine, Bricanyl

AsthmaHaler (epinephrine)
AsthmaNefrin (epincphriue)
Beta-2 Bronkometer
  isoetharine
Brethaire (terbutaline)
Brethine (terbutaline)
Bricanyl (terbutaline)
Bronitin Mist (epinephrine)
Bronkaid Mist (epinephrine)
Bronkephrine
  ethylnorepinephrine
Bronkosol (isoetharine)
Dey-Dose Isoproterenol
Dey-Dose (epinephrine)
Dey-Lute (isoetharine)
Disorine (isoetharine)
Dispos-a-Med Isoetharine
Dispos-a-Med Isoproterenol
Efed II (ephedrine)
Ephedrine Sulfate (ephedrine)
Isuprel (isoproterenol)
Maxair (pirbuterol)
Medihaler-Epi (epinephrine)
Medihaler-Iso (isoproterenol)
Metaprel (metaproterenol)
microNefrin (epinephrine)
Primatene Mist (epinephrine)
Proventil (albuterol)
S-2 Inhalant (epinephrine)
Sus-Phrine (epinephrine)
Tornalate (bitolterol)
Vapo-Iso (isoproterenol)
Vaponefrin (epinephrine)
Ventolin (albuterol)

Asthma Drugs (theophyllines):

By generic name
aminophylline (Somophyllin)
dyphylline (Dilor, Lufyllin)
oxtriphylline (Choledyl)
theophylline

By brand name
Aerolate (theophylline)
Bronkaid (theophylline)
Bronkodyl (theophylline)
Choledyl (oxtriphylline)

Aerolate, Bronkodyl, Bronkaid
Constant-T, Elixophyllin
Marax, Mudrane, Primatene
Quibron, Respbid, Slo-bid
Slo-Phylline, T-PHYL, Tedral
Theo-24, Theo-Dur
Theo-Organidin, Theobid
Theolair, Theospan-SR
Theostat 80, Uniphyl

Constant-T (theophylline)
Dilor (dyphylline)
Elixophyllin (theophylline)
Lufyllin (dyphylline)
Marax (theophylline)
Mudrane (theophylline)
Primatene (theophylline)
Quibron (theophylline)
Respbid (theophylline)
Slo-bid (theophylline)
Slo-Phylline (theophylline)
Somophyllin (aminophylline)
T-PHYL (theophylline)
Tedral (theophylline)
Theo-24 (theophylline)
Theo-Dur (theophylline)
Theo-Organidin
  theophylline
Theobid (theophylline)
Theolair (theophylline)
Theospan-SR (theophylline)
Theostat 80 (theophylline)
Uniphyl (theophylline)

CAFFEINE

e.g., coffee, colas, tea
cold/cough products
menstrual discomfort products
pain products
(Read product labels)

DECONGESTANTS, NASAL

Nasal decongestants (used in cold/cough products) help reverse nasal congestion by shrinking swollen blood vessels in the nasal mucosa, allowing easier breathing and better nasal and sinus drainage. (Check labels on multi-ingredient cold/cough products—many contain nasal decongestants.)

ORAL *(by mouth):*

By generic name
ephedrine
phenylephrine
phenylpropanolamine
pseudoephedrine
By brand name
  Afrinol
  Allerest No Drowsiness
  Dorcol Children's
    Decongestant
  Dristan Maximum Strength
  Fiogesic, Entex, Naldegesic
  Novafed, Ornex, Propagest
  Sinarest No Drowsiness
  Sine-Aid, Sine-Off
  Sinus Excedrin, Sinutab
  St. Joseph Cold Tablets
    for Children
  Sudafed, Tylenol
  Sinus, Ursinus

TOPICAL *(nasal drops, spray, inhaler):*

By generic name
ephedrine
epinephrine
naphazoline
oxymetazoline
phenylephrine
propylhexedrine
tetrahydrozoline
xylometazoline
By brand name
  4-Way, Adrenalin Chloride
  Afrin, Alconefrin, Allerest
  12-Hour Nasal, Benzedrex
  inhaler, Coricidin Nasal
  Doktors, Dristan, Duration
  Efedron Nasal
  Neo-Synephrine, Nostril,
  Otrivin, Privine, Rhinall
  Nostrilla, NTZ, Sinarest,
  Sinex, Twice-A-Day
  Tyzine, Vatronol
  Vicks inhaler

METHYLPHENIDATE (Ritalin)

Methylphenidate is used for Attention Deficit Disorders (ADDs) in children and for narcolepsy (uncontrollable desire to sleep). Unlabeled uses include treatment of depression in the elderly and in cancer and post-stroke patients.

PEMOLINE (Cylert)

Pemoline is used for Attention Deficit Disorders (ADDs) in children; unlabeled uses include narcolepsy (uncontrollable desire to sleep) and excessive daytime sleepiness.

Diseases/Disorders and the Drugs Used to Treat Them

This section presents a brief overview of common diseases/disorders and the drugs used to treat them. Many of the drugs/drug classes listed appear in the index. Look there to find an interaction number, then see the text for a list of individual generic and brand names.

ALLERGIES

ANXIETY DISORDERS

ARTHRITIS

ASTHMA (BRONCHIAL)

COMMON COLD

DEPRESSION

DIABETES

EPILEPSY AND SEIZURE DISORDERS

HEART DISORDERS

HIGH BLOOD PRESSURE

INDIGESTION

INFECTIONS, MICROBIAL

INSOMNIA

MENTAL ILLNESS (PSYCHOSIS)

OVERWEIGHT

PAIN

THYROID DISORDERS

ULCERS (GASTRIC AND DUODENAL)

ALLERGIES

Allergic reactions are usually caused by the body's release of *histamine* in response to invasion by an allergen. Some people are more susceptible to allergens than others.

A common allergy syndrome is *Seasonal Allergic Rhinitis* (SAR), also known as hay fever or pollinosis. It is caused by ragweed, grass pollen, and tree pollens, and recurs annually during the pollinating season. Individuals suffering symptoms throughout the year may have what is termed *perennial allergic rhinitis* and are susceptible to allergens in house dust, mold and fungus spores, feathers, talcum powder, and animal dander.

Symptoms include uncontrollable sneezing attacks, itching, runny or stuffy nose, itchy and watery eyes, sensitivity to light, headache and irritability, insomnia, and lack of appetite.

Drugs Used for Allergies

Antihistamines
Corticosteroids

Antihistamines work by displacing histamine from its binding sites in body cells.
Corticosteroids reduce swelling and inflammation.

ANXIETY DISORDERS

Feelings of anxiety and apprehension due to an environmental event such as attending a job interview are considered normal. On the other hand, anxiety disorders such as chronic panic attacks result from neurologic dysfunctions that may have a genetic component.

Drugs used are called *antianxiety agents. Benzodiazepines* are the type most widely used.

Drug Used for Anxiety

benzodiazepines
non-benzodiazepines
  buspirone
  chlormezanone
  doxepin
  droperidol
  hydroxyzine
  meprobamate

ARTHRITIS

Arthritis is a disease causing inflammation of the joints. Two major types are osteoarthritis and rheumatoid arthritis.

Osteoarthritis or degenerative arthritis worsens with aging as bone cartilage wears down. Pain and inflammation are aggravated by weather changes and activity.

The debilitating effects of *rheumatoid arthritis* can occur at any age, causing swollen, painful joints and eventually joint deformities.

Drugs Used for Arthritis

corticosteroids
NSAIDs (nonsteroidal antiinflammatory drugs)

Both *corticosteroids* and *nonsteroidal antiinflammatory drugs* (NSAIDs) reduce swelling and inflammation.

ASTHMA (BRONCHIAL)

Bronchial asthma causes difficulty in breathing due to constriction of airways and bronchioles in the lungs. The asthmatic reaction, depending on the sufferer, may be associated with certain drugs, foods and food preservatives, stress, exercise, respiratory tract infections, or inhaled particles such as pollen, mold, or dust.

Drugs Used for Bronchial Asthma

corticosteroids
sympathomimetics
theophyllines

Corticosteroids counter the allergic and inflammatory reaction that causes constricted air passages.

Both *sympathomimetics* and *theophyllines* are bronchodilators which open constricted air passages.

COMMON COLD

The most widespread human ailment is the common cold, which hits each person an average of twice a year. A cold is likely to be caught during times of temperature change—in early fall, just after midwinter, and in early spring.

Most colds are caused by viruses called rhinoviruses and coronaviruses that spread by sneezing, coughing, and physical contact.

The onset of a cold can be abrupt. Initial symptoms may be a dry, itchy throat and nose, headache or body aches, or a cough. Children usually have a fever. Secretions increase, the nose runs and becomes congested, the eyes water, and nasal irritation causes sneezing.

Currently there is no cure for the cold. The body's natural defenses will restore normalcy within a few days.

Drugs Used for Common Cold

Antihistamines
Decongestants, nasal

Antihistamines have a drying effect, which counters symptoms caused by hypersecretion, such as runny nose and watery, itchy eyes. The earlier an antihistamine is taken, the more effective it is.

Nasal decongestants reverse nasal congestion by shrinking swollen blood vessels in the nasal mucosa, allowing easier breathing and better nasal and sinus drainage.

DEPRESSION

Millions of people suffer the debilitating effects of clinical depression. Sufferers of depressive illness have feelings—beyond their conscious control—of hopelessness, worthlessness, and despair.

We are coming more and more to recognize that the root causes of depression—and other so-called emotional or mental disorders—stem from biologic causes or predispositions. These disorders are physical disorders in the same way that asthma and diabetes are. They need carry no stigma.

The most successful treatment has been with the use of *antidepressant drugs*. These drugs are believed to work by increasing the amounts of brain neurotransmitter chemicals such as serotonin or norepinephrine, and in many cases they alleviate the adverse symptoms of depression.

Drugs Used for Depression

antidepressants (cyclic-type)
antidepressants (MAOI-type)

DIABETES

Diabetes mellitus is a disease in which either the pancreas gland fails to produce enough insulin or the body cannot use insulin properly. Insulin is a hormone which transports sugar from the blood into body cells needing it for energy.

In diabetes, sugar remains in the bloodstream (and appears in the urine) instead of being taken in and used by body cells. Denied sugar, the cells must burn more than ordinary amounts of fats and proteins for fuel. This excessive breakdown of fats and proteins releases acid waste products into the blood.

Untreated or poorly controlled diabetes causes long-term adverse effects and may result in a metabolic crisis and diabetic coma.

Symptoms of diabetes include excessive appetite (the body recognizes its increased need for fuel); large urine output; excessive thirst (the body must replace fluid lost through urination); weakness, lethargy, drowsiness; and weight loss.

Some diabetics with non-insulin-dependent Type II diabetes can be treated by diet and weight control alone. Some require oral medication. Those with insulin-dependent Type 1 diabetes (also called juvenile-onset diabetes) may require daily insulin injections.

Both oral pills and insulin cause a lowering of the blood sugar level. The pills work either by stimulating the pancreas to produce more insulin or by enhancing the body's ability to use it. Injection provides a direct replacement for the body's own lack of insulin.

Drugs Used for Diabetes

sulfonylureas (also called oral hypoglycemics)
insulin

EPILEPSY AND SEIZURE DISORDERS

An epileptic seizure may result from a "short-circuit" in a part of the brain, a nerve discharge which spills over to other nerves in that area, sometimes causing spasmodic limb and body movements and alterations in consciousness.

Grand mal epilepsy is the seizure disorder most associated with epilepsy. The seizure—often presaged by a distinct smell or odor or some other sensation—begins suddenly and causes jerking of the arms and legs, chewing or gnawing of the teeth, and arching of the neck. The seizure usually runs its course and subsides. The main danger to the victim is from falling, biting the tongue, or choking on saliva or vomit.

Petit mal or "absence" seizure is a sudden loss of awareness of the surroundings. The sufferer may stare blankly ahead for a few seconds, often making random, purposeless movements.

Psychomotor seizures originate in the temporal lobe of the brain and cause a variety of effects, usually followed by amnesia about the attack. Psychomotor seizures may presage a grand mal episode.

Flashing lights—such as from a flickering TV screen or computer video game—may precipitate seizures in seizure-prone individuals.

Anticonvulsant drugs are used to prevent seizures. Dilantin (phenytoin) is the most widely used anticonvulsant drug.

Drugs Used for Epilepsy and Seizure Disorders

anticonvulsants:
  carbamazepine
  clonazepam
  clorazepate
  diazepam
  ethosuximide
  ethotoin
  mephenytoin
  methsuximide
  paramethadione
  phenacemide
  phensuximide
  phenytoin
  primidone
  trimethadione
  valproic acid

HEART DISORDERS

The most common disorders of the heart are angina, heart beat irregularities (cardiac arrhythmias), and congestive heart failure.

Angina pain results when the heart itself does not receive enough oxygen-carrying blood. This happens when blood flow through coronary (heart) arteries becomes impeded. The discomfort may be brought on in situations demanding more work by the heart, such as exertion and stress.

Heart beat irregularities are disturbances in the heart's normal rhythm. The various types include fibrillation, flutter, palpitation (skipped beats), premature beat, and paroxysmal tachycardia (episodes of very rapid heart beat).

Congestive heart failure occurs when the heart fails to pump blood out as fast as it comes in. This causes blood to back up and overfill the lungs, resulting in shortness of breath and accumulation of fluid in body tissues.

Drugs Used for Heart Disorders

ACE inhibitors
angina drugs
anti-arrhythmics
  digoxin
  quinidine
  disopyramide
  procainamide
  tocainide
beta blockers
calcium blockers
  diltiazem
  nicardipine
  nifedipine
  nimodipine
  verapamil
digitalis
  digitoxin
  digoxin
diuretics

ACE inhibitors are used for congestive heart failure and high blood pressure.

Angina drugs relieve angina pain by improving the supply of blood and oxygen to the heart.

Anti-arrhythmics restore irregular heart beats to normal rhythm.

Beta blockers are used for angina pain, irregular heart beats, and high blood pressure. Some are used to prevent migraine headaches and to relieve the physical manifestations of "stage fright."

Calcium blockers are used for angina pain, irregular heart beats, and high blood pressure.

Digitalis improves the strength and efficiency of the heart and is used for congestive heart failure and heart beat irregularities.

Diuretics remove excess body fluid and are used for congestive heart failure and high blood pressure.

HIGH BLOOD PRESSURE

High blood pressure, or *essential hypertension,* left untreated increases the risk of heart attack and stroke. Since the condition may cause no obvious symptoms, it is usually discovered by a routine physical examination.

A normal blood pressure reading for a young adult is approximately 120/80. 120 is the *systolic* pressure and 80 is the *diastolic* pressure. The systolic number indicates the pumping pressure in the arteries; the diastolic number, the resting pressure.

Treatment for high blood pressure is usually begun when the diastolic pressure consistently exceeds ninety (90) in readings taken over several days.

The physician may first recommend nondrug measures to lower blood pressure: dietary salt restriction (salt causes the body to retain fluid, thereby adding to blood volume and increasing pressure within the vessels), weight reduction, and quitting smoking. If satisfactory results aren't achieved, drug treatment is begun.

Drugs Used for High Blood Pressure

ACE inhibitors
beta blockers
calcium blockers
  diltiazem
  nicardipine

    nifedipine
    nimodipine
    verapamil
  diuretics
  nerve blockers
    clonidine
    guanabenz
    guanethidine
    methyldopa
    prazosin
    reserpine
  vasodilators
    hydralazine
    loniten

ACE inhibitors work by preventing the conversion of a chemical released by the kidney into a form that raises blood pressure.

Beta blockers lower blood pressure in several ways such as slowing heart rate and decreasing the amount of blood pumped per beat.

Calcium blockers lower blood pressure and also are used for angina pain and irregular heart beats.

Diuretics lower blood pressure by removing excess body fluid and also may be used for congestive heart failure.

Nerve blockers block the nerve impulses that raise blood pressure.

Vasodilators lower blood pressure by relaxing and dilating blood vessels.

INDIGESTION

Everyone suffers now and then from the discomforts of indigestion, also called *dyspepsia*. It can be caused by overindulgence in food and drink, poor chewing habits (chewing is the first step in digestion), swallowing air while eating, or the use of stomach-irritating drugs.

Symptoms may include heartburn, sour or acid stomach, cramps, nausea, and excessive gas. Most cases of indigestion are uncomplicated and respond readily to treatment with nonprescription antacids. *Antacids* work by helping to neutralize excess hydrochloric acid in stomach fluids.

Drugs Used for Indigestion

  antacids

INFECTIONS, MICROBIAL

Microbial (usually bacterial) infections include bronchitis, pneumonia, strep throat, tonsillitis, cystitis or urinary tract (bladder and kidney) infections, ear infections, sinusitis, syphilis, gonorrhea, vaginitis, cholera, Rocky Mountain Spotted Fever, chancre sores, conjunctivitis of the eye, and intestinal amebiasis.

Many people think that antibiotics are prescribed for colds or the flu. They may indeed be prescribed at the same time but only to ward off a secondary microbial infection such as strep throat, not for the cold or flu, which are caused by viruses.

Drugs Used for Infections

    antibiotics:
      aminoglycosides
      antibiotics, quinolone
      cephalosporins
      chloroamphenicol
      erythromycin
      metronidazole
      penicillin
      tetracycline
      troleandomycin

INSOMNIA

Almost everyone experiences occasional insomnia (sleeplessness), especially during periods of unusual tension or upset. Physicians may prescribe a sedative or sleep inducer for short-term use.

Drugs Used for Insomnia

    antihistamines (nonprescription):
      diphenhydramine
      doxylamine
    barbiturates
    benzodiazepines

non-barbiturates:
  chloral hydrate
  ethchlorvynol
  ethinamate
  glutethimide
  methyprylon
  paraldehyde

MENTAL ILLNESS (PSYCHOSIS)

A severe mental illness (psychosis) such as schizophrenia, paranoia, or manic-depressive disorder results from a disorder or dysfunction of the brain areas governing thought and behavior.

In *schizophrenia* the sufferer exhibits an inability to relate to other people, and usually has delusions, hallucinations, and a loss of contact with reality.

Paranoia causes one to believe it is his supreme purpose to undertake some irrational (to him totally rational and justified) act, and that others are trying to prevent him from completing his self-appointed mission.

In *manic-depressive disorder,* the mood swings to and fro like a pendulum—from abject depression to unbridled optimism—totally out of proportion to the situation.

Until research uncovers the specific genetic and physical causes for this type of illness, treatment is aimed at controlling the symptoms so that the patient can function in society without harming himself and others.

The drugs used to treat psychoses are called *antipsychotics*. There are three types.

Drugs Used for Mental Illness

lithium
phenothiazines
non-phenothiazines:
  chlorprothixene
  haloperidol
  loxapine
  molindone
  thiothixene

OVERWEIGHT

With today's emphasis on looks and fitness, many overweight people turn to *appetite suppressants,* or diet pills, to help them shed a few pounds—or a lot of pounds in some cases. By curbing the appetite, these drugs serve as temporary help while one tries to develop the proper eating habits needed over the long term. It must not be overlooked that genetic predisposition plays a role in body weight.

Drugs Used for Weight Loss

appetite suppressants

PAIN

Pain can be a symptom associated with almost any ailment. Though sometimes excruciating, it is invaluable as both a diagnostic aid and a sensory warning signal that something is wrong.

Pain may be characterized as superficial, visceral, or somatic. *Superficial* pain comes from skin or mucous membranes and is usually sharp and localized. *Visceral* pain is deeper, originating in an organ system such as the stomach or kidneys. *Somatic* pain comes from skeletal muscles, joints, or ligaments and is usually dull, aching, and not sharply localized—for example, headache, toothache, and arthritic and muscular aches. Pain relieving drugs are classified as narcotics and non-narcotics.

Drugs Used for Pain

narcotics (eg, codeine, meperidine)
non-narcotics:
  acetaminophen
  NSAIDs
    (Nonsteroidal antiinflammatory drugs)
  propoxyphene
  salicylates (e.g., aspirin)

THYROID DISORDERS

The thyroid gland, located in the neck, plays an important role in body metabolism.

A person with *hyperthyroidism* produces too much thyroid hormone, which causes overactivity, anxiety, hand tremors, weight loss, and perhaps bulging of the eyes.

Hypothyroidism, or lack of enough thyroid hormone, may cause the thyroid gland to enlarge in an effort to produce more hormone, resulting in a *goiter.* Associated symptoms include weight gain, dry coarse hair, and puffiness of the face. Newborn infants with a congenital thyroid deficiency suffer from what is called *cretinism.* In adults, severe cases of hypothyroidism are called *myxedema.*

Hypothyroidism and goiter are treated with replacement thyroid drugs. Hyperthyroidism is treated with antithyroid drugs such as propylthiouracil and methimazole.

Drugs Used for Thyroid Disorders (hypothyroidism)

thyroid

ULCERS (GASTRIC AND DUODENAL)

A gastric ulcer is an erosion in the stomach lining. A duodenal ulcer occurs in the duodenum (the first part of the small intestine, into which the stomach content empties). The usual symptom of an ulcer is pain or "heartburn" in the upper abdomen or lower chest, especially after eating irritating foods or drinking alcohol or coffee. Bleeding from an ulcer may cause the stool to look black or tarry, and general weakness and fatigue may occur due to loss of blood.

Patients should determine for themselves what foods (if any) cause discomfort and then avoid them. Nevertheless, it's still a sound idea for all ulcer patients to avoid alcohol, coffee, colas, and other beverages containing caffeine, which increases stomach acid secretion.

Drugs Used for Ulcers

antacids
anticholinergics
histamine H2 antagonists
  cimetidine
  famotidine
  nizatidine
  ranitidine
misoprostol
omeprazole
sucralfate

Antacids work by neutralizing the acid secreted by the stomach.

Anticholinergics reduce acid secretion and reduce "motility" or movement of the smooth muscle in the stomach and intestine.

Histamine H2 antagonists and the drugs *misoprostol* and *omeprazole* inhibit stomach acid secretion.

Sulcralfate works by forming a sort of "bandage" around the ulcer, protecting it from irritating acid.

A-Z
Drug
Interactions

1.   ↓ **ACE Inhibitors**   **food**
     captopril (Capoten)

     Severity: ●●○
     Probability: ●○○

     USES: Captopril is used for high blood pressure and heart failure.
     EFFECT: The effect of captopril may be decreased. (Food does not seem to affect other ACE inhibitors.)
     RESULT: The condition treated may not be properly controlled.
     WHAT TO DO: Take captopril an hour before meals.

2.   ↓ **ACE Inhibitors**   **Indomethacin (Indocin)**
     captopril (Capoten)
     lisinopril (Prinivil, Zestril)
     enalapril (Vasotec)
     ramipril (Altace)

     Severity: ●●○
     Probability: ●●○

     USES: ACE inhibitors are used for high blood pressure and heart failure. Indomethacin is a nonsteroidal antiinflammatory drug (NSAID) used for pain and inflammation in severe arthritic-type conditions.
     EFFECT: The effect of the ACE inhibitor to lower blood pressure may be decreased.
     RESULT: The blood pressure may not be properly controlled.
     WHAT TO DO: Monitor blood pressure. Replace the ACE inhibitor with an alternative medication or stop indomethacin as warranted.

3.   **acetaminophen**   **alcohol (ethanol)**
     Anacin-3, Datril, Excedrin,   beer, liquor, wine
     Percogesic, Tempra, Tylenol

     Severity: ●●○
     Probability: ●○○

     USES: Acetaminophen is used for pain and fever.
     RESULT: Acetaminophen-caused liver damage may be increased by chronic use of alcoholic beverages.
     WHAT TO DO: Avoid either chronic, excessive drinking or regular use of acetaminophen. (Note: Several over-the-counter combination products for pain/fever and cold/cough also contain acetaminophen—read product labels.)

4. ↓ **acetaminophen**   **phenytoin (Dilantin)**
    Anacin-3, Datril, Excedrin,   ethotoin (Peganone)
    Percogesic, Tempra, Tylenol   mephenytoin (Mesantoin)

    Severity: ●●○
    Probability: ●○○

USES: Acetaminophen is used for pain and fever. Phenytoin is an anticonvulsant used for seizure disorders such as epilepsy.

RESULT: The risk of acetaminophen-caused liver damage may be increased; also, the therapeutic action of acetaminophen may be decreased so that pain or fever is not properly controlled.

WHAT TO DO: Do not exceed the recommended dose of either drug. (Note: Several over-the-counter combination products for pain/fever and cold/cough also contain acetaminophen—read product labels.)

5. ↓ **acetaminophen**   **sulfinpyrazone**
    Anacin-3, Datril, Excedrin,   **(Anturane)**
    Percogesic, Tempra, Tylenol

    Severity: ●●○
    Probability: ●○○

USES: Acetaminophen is used for pain and fever. Sulfinpyrazone is used for gouty arthritis.

RESULT: The risk of acetaminophen-caused liver damage may be increased; also, the therapeutic action of acetaminophen may be decreased so that pain or fever is not properly controlled.

WHAT TO DO: Do not exceed the recommended dose of either drug. (Note: Several over-the-counter combination products for pain/fever and cold/cough also contain acetaminophen—read product labels.)

6. ↑ **alcohol (ethanol)**   ↑ **barbiturates**
    beer, liquor, wine   amobarbital (Amytal)
                                           aprobarbital (Alurate)
                                           butabarbital (Butisol)
                                           butalbital
                                           mephobarbital (Mebaral)
                                           pentobarbital (Nembutal)
                                           phenobarbital
                                           primidone (Mysoline)
                                           secobarbital (Seconal)
                                           talbutal (Lotusate)

Severity: ●●●
Probability: ●●●

USES: Barbiturates are used as sedatives or sleep inducers; phenobarbital and primidone are used in seizure disorders such as epilepsy.

EFFECT: "Add-on" depressant effects of each drug.

RESULT: Increased risk of excessive central nervous system depression with symptoms such as drowsiness, dizziness, loss of muscle coordination and alertness; in severe cases, failure of blood circulation and breathing functions causing coma and death.

WHAT TO DO: Avoid this combination.

7. ↑ **alcohol (ethanol)**
   beer, liquor, wine

   ↑ **benzodiazepines**
   alprazolam (Xanax)
   chlordiazepoxide (Librium)
   clonazepam (Klonopin)
   clorazepate (Tranxene)
   diazepam (Valium)
   estazolam (ProSom)
   flurazepam (Dalmane)
   halazepam (Paxipam)
   lorazepam (Ativan)
   midazolam (Versed)
   oxazepam (Serax)
   prazepam (Centrax)
   quazepam (Doral)
   temazepam (Restoril)
   triazolam (Halcion)

Severity: ●●○
Probability: ●●●

USES: Benzodiazepines are used for anxiety; some are used to induce sleep.

EFFECT: "Add-on" depressant effects of each drug.

RESULT: Increased risk of excessive central nervous system depression with symptoms such as drowsiness, dizziness, loss of muscle coordination and mental alertness; in severe cases, failure of blood circulation and breathing functions causing coma and death.

WHAT TO DO: Avoid this combination.

8.   alcohol (ethanol)   **cephalosporins**
beer, liquor, wine   cefamandole (Mandol)
                                            cefonicid(Monocid)
                                            cefoperazone (Cefobid)
                                            ceforanide (Precef)
                                            cefotetan (Cefotan)
                                            moxalactam (Moxam)

Severity: ●●○
Probability: ●●○

USES: Cephalosporins are antibiotics related to penicillin and are used for microbial infections.

RESULT: Disulfiram-type reaction (flushing, nausea, vomiting, dizziness, shortness of breath, severe headache, visual disturbances, heart palpitations, possible unconsciousness). This effect may occur immediately or several days after taking this drug combination.

WHAT TO DO: Avoid this combination.

9.   ↑ alcohol (ethanol)   **↑ chloral hydrate (Noctec)**

beer, liquor, wine

Severity: ●●○
Probability: ●●●

USES: Chloral Hydrate is used to induce sleep.

EFFECT: "Add-on" depressant effects of each drug.

RESULT: Increased risk of excessive central nervous system depression with symptoms such as drowsiness, dizziness, loss of muscle coordination and mental alertness; in severe cases, failure of blood circulation and breathing functions causing coma and death.

WHAT TO DO: Avoid this combination.

10. ↑ alcohol (ethanol)   **cimetidine (Tagamet)**
beer, liquor, wine

Severity: ●●○
Probability: ●○○

USES: Cimetidine is used for gastric and duodenal ulcers.

EFFECT: The body's absorption of alcohol may be increased.

RESULT: Increased risk of alcoholic intoxication with symptoms such as drowsiness, dizziness, loss of muscle coordination and mental alertness.

WHAT TO DO: Avoid this combination or drink alcoholic beverages with care.

11.   alcohol (ethanol)   disulfiram (Antabuse)
       beer, liquor, wine

    Severity: ●●●
Probability: ●●●

USES: Disulfiram is prescribed to deter ingestion of alcoholic beverages.

EFFECT: The "disulfiram reaction."

RESULT: Flushing, nausea, vomiting, dizziness, shortness of breath, severe headache, visual disturbances, heart palpitations, possible unconsciousness.

WHAT TO DO: Avoid this combination.

12.   alcohol (ethanol)   furazolidone (Furoxone)
       beer, liquor, wine

    Severity: ●●○
Probability: ●●○

USES: Furazolidone is used for bacterial and protozoal diarrhea and enteritis (inflammation of the intestines).

RESULT: Disulfiram-type reaction (flushing, nausea, vomiting, dizziness, shortness of breath, severe headache, visual disturbances, heart palpitations, possible unconsciousness).

WHAT TO DO: Avoid this combination.

13. ↑ alcohol (ethanol)   ↑ glutethimide (Doriden)
       beer, liquor, wine

    Severity: ●●○
Probability: ●○○

USES: Glutethimide is used to induce sleep.

EFFECT: "Add-on" depressant effects of each drug.

RESULT: Increased risk of excessive central nervous system depression with symptoms such as drowsiness, dizziness, loss of muscle coordination and mental alertness; in severe cases, failure of blood circulation and breathing functions causing coma and death.

WHAT TO DO: Avoid this combination.

14. ↑ **alcohol (ethanol)**   ↑ **meprobamate**
     beer, liquor, wine   Equanil, Miltown

    Severity: ●●○
    Probability: ●●○

USES: Meprobamate is used for anxiety disorders.

EFFECT: "Add-on" depressant effects of each drug.

RESULT: Increased risk of excessive central nervous system depression with symptoms such as drowsiness, dizziness, loss of muscle coordination and mental alertness; in severe cases, failure of blood circulation and breathing functions causing coma and death.

WHAT TO DO: Avoid this combination.

15. ↑ **alcohol (ethanol)**   **metoclopramide**
     beer, liquor, wine   **(Reglan)**

    Severity: ●●○
    Probability: ●○○

USES: Metoclopramide is used for gastroesophageal reflux (a backward flow of stomach contents) and, in higher doses, for preventing vomiting associated with some types of cancer chemotherapy.

EFFECT: The body's absorption of alcohol may be increased.

RESULT: Increased risk of alcoholic intoxication with symptoms such as drowsiness, dizziness, loss of muscle coordination and mental alertness.

WHAT TO DO: Avoid this combination or drink alcoholic beverages with care.

16. **alcohol (ethanol)**   **metronidazole**
     beer, liquor, wine   Flagyl, Metryl, Protostat

    Severity: ●●○
    Probability: ●○○

USES: Metronidazole is used for trichomoniasis, a venereal disease.

RESULT: Disulfiram-type reaction (flushing, nausea, vomiting, dizziness, shortness of breath, severe headache, visual disturbances, heart palpitations, possible unconsciousness).

WHAT TO DO: Avoid this combination.

17. ↑ **alcohol (ethanol)**   ↑ **phenothiazines**
        beer, liquor, wine   acetophenazine (Tindal)
                                                                    chlorpromazine (Thorazine)
                                                                    fluphenazine (Permitil,
                                                                      Prolixin)
                                                                    mesoridazine (Serentil)
                                                                    perphenazine (Trilafon)
                                                                    prochlorperazine (Compazine)
                                                                    promazine (Sparine)
                                                                    promethazine (Phenergan)
                                                                    thioridazine (Mellaril)
                                                                    trifluoperazine (Stelazine)

   Severity: ●●○
   Probability: ●●○

USES: Phenothiazines are antipsychotic drugs used for brain disorders such as schizophrenia, paranoia, and manic-depressive disorder.

EFFECT: "Add-on" depressant effects of each drug.

RESULT: Increased risk of excessive central nervous system depression with symptoms such as drowsiness, dizziness, loss of muscle coordination and mental alertness; in severe cases, failure of blood circulation and breathing functions causing coma and death; also, an increased chance of phenothiazine-caused brain dysfunctions.

WHAT TO DO: Avoid this combination.

18. **alcohol (ethanol)**   **procarbazine (Matulane)**
        beer, liquor, wine

   Severity: ●○○
   Probability: ●○○

USES: Procarbazine is used for Hodgkin's disease.

RESULT: Facial flushing.

WHAT TO DO: Avoid drinking alcoholic beverages.

19. **allopurinol (Zyloprim)**   **ACE inhibitors**
                                                                    captopril (Capoten)
                                                                    lisinopril (Prinivil, Zestril)
                                                                    enalapril (Vasotec)
                                                                    ramipril (Altace)

   Severity: ●●●
   Probability: ●○○

USES: Allopurinol is used for gout and in certain types of cancer therapy. ACE inhibitors are used for high blood pressure and heart failure.

RESULT: Increased risk of a hypersensitivity reaction.

WHAT TO DO: If hypersensitivity (severe allergic reaction with symptoms such as fever, skin rashes, muscle and joint pain) develops, stop both drugs and contact your physician immediately.

20. ↓ **antibiotics, quinolone**

ciprofloxacin (Cipro)
enoxacin (Comprecin)
norfloxacin (Noroxin)
ofloxacin (Floxin)

antacids

aluminum-magnesium
  hydroxides
  eg: Delcid, Di-Gel, Gelusil,
  Maalox, Mylanta, Riopan

Severity: ●●○
Probability: ●○○

USES: Quinolone antibiotics are used to treat a broad range of microbial infections. Antacids are used for stomach problems associated with too much stomach acid.

EFFECT: The effects of the antibiotic may be decreased.

RESULT: The infection treated may not be properly controlled.

WHAT TO DO: Take the antacid at least 6 hours before or 2 hours after the antibiotic.

21. ↓ **antibiotics, quinolone**

ciprofloxacin (Cipro)
enoxacin (Comprecin)
norfloxacin (Noroxin)
ofloxacin (Floxin)

iron

ferrous fumarate
ferrous gluconate
ferrous sulfate
iron polysaccharide
Brand names:
  Caltrate, Chromagen, Feosol
  Feostat, Ferancee, Fergon
  Fero-Folic-500, Fero-Grad-50
  Ferralet, Ferro-Sequel
  Fosfree, Hemocyte, Hytinic
  Iberet, Ircon, Iromin-G
  Mission Prenatal, Mol-Iron
  Natalins Rx, Poly-Vi-Flor
  Pramet FA, Pramilet FA
  Simron, Slow Fe, Stuartinic
  Trinsicon, Zenate

Severity: ●●○
Probability: ●○○

USES: Quinolone antibiotics are used to treat a broad range of microbial infections. The mineral iron is an essential component of hemoglobin in the blood.
EFFECT: The effects of the antibiotic may be decreased.
RESULT: The infection treated may not be properly controlled.
WHAT TO DO: Avoid this combination if feasible.

22. ↓ **antibiotics, quinolone**   **sucralfate (Carafate)**
    ciprofloxacin (Cipro)
    enoxacin (Comprecin)
    norfloxacin (Noroxin)
    ofloxacin (Floxin)

    Severity: ●●○
    Probability: ●○○

USES: Quinolone antibiotics are used to treat a broad range of microbial infections. Sucralfate is used for stomach ulcers.
EFFECT: The effects of the antibiotic may be decreased.
RESULT: The infection treated may not be properly controlled.
WHAT TO DO: Avoid this combination if feasible.

23. ↑ **antidepressants, tricyclic**   **cimetidine (Tagamet)**
    amitriptyline (Elavil, Endep)
    amoxapine (Asendin)
    clomipramine (Anafranil)
    desipramine
      Norpramin, Pertofrane
    doxepin (Adapin, Sinequan)
    imipramine (Tofranil)
    nortriptyline
      Aventyl, Pamelor
    protriptyline (Vivactil)
    trimipramine (Surmontil)

    Severity: ●●○
    Probability: ●●○

USES: Tricyclic antidepressants are prescribed for clinical depression. Cimetidine is used for gastric and duodenal ulcers.

EFFECT: The adverse effects of the antidepressant may be increased.

RESULT: Symptoms include lethargy, drowsiness, loss of coordination, blurry vision, dry mouth, rapid heart beat, confusion.

WHAT TO DO: Monitor antidepressant blood levels and symptoms, and adjust the dose as needed. Option: use ranitidine (Zantac), which appears not to interact, in place of cimetidine.

24. ↑ antidepressants, tricyclic   fluoxetine (Prozac)
     amitriptyline (Elavil, Endep)
     amoxapine (Asendin)
     clomipramine (Anafranil)
     desipramine
        Norpramin, Pertofrane
     doxepin (Adapin, Sinequan)
     imipramine (Tofranil)
     nortriptyline
        Aventyl, Pamelor
     protriptyline (Vivactil)
     trimipramine (Surmontil)

     Severity: ●●○
Probability: ●○○

USES: Tricyclic antidepressants are prescribed for clinical depression. Fluoxetine is a non-tricyclic antidepressant prescribed for clinical depression.

EFFECT: The adverse effects of the tricyclic antidepressant may be increased.

RESULT: Symptoms include lethargy, drowsiness, loss of coordination, blurry vision, dry mouth, rapid heart beat, confusion.

WHAT TO DO: Monitor antidepressant blood levels and symptoms, and adjust the dose as needed.

25.   antidepressants, tricyclic   MAO inhibitors
       amitriptyline (Elavil, Endep)   isocarboxazid (Marplan)
       amoxapine (Asendin)   pargyline (Eutonyl)
       clomipramine (Anafranil)   phenelzine (Nardil)
       desipramine   tranylcypromine (Parnate)
          Norpramin, Pertofrane
       doxepin (Adapin, Sinequan)
       imipramine (Tofranil)

nortriptyline
  Aventyl, Pamelor
protriptyline (Vivactil)
trimipramine (Surmontil)

Severity: ●●●
Probability: ●○○

USES: Both types of drugs are antidepressants used to treat clinical depression.

RESULT: This combination can cause severe excitability, headache, fever, rapid heart beat, low blood pressure, seizures, coma, and in severe cases, death.

WHAT TO DO: Avoid this combination if possible or start them together at lower doses and increase the doses cautiously. Stop both drugs if adverse effects appear.

26. ↑ **appetite suppressants**   **furazolidone (Furoxone)**
      amphetamine
      benzphetamine (Didrex)
      dextroamphetamine
        Biphetamine, Dexedrine
      diethylpropion (Tenuate)
      fenfluramine (Pondimin)
      mazindol (Sanorex)
      methamphetamine (Desoxyn)
      phenmetrazine (Preludin)
      phentermine (Ionamin)

Severity: ●●○
Probability: ●○○

USES: Appetite suppressants are used as short-term therapy in a weight loss program. Furazolidone is used for bacterial and protozoal diarrhea and enteritis (inflammation of the intestines).

EFFECT: The adverse effects of the appetite suppressant may be increased.

RESULT: Possible dangerous rise in blood pressure with symptoms such as severe headache, fever, visual disturbances, nervousness, confusion which, in severe cases, may be followed by brain hemorrhage and stroke.

WHAT TO DO: Watch for adverse symptoms and lower the dose of the appetite suppressant as needed.

27. ↑ **appetite suppressants**   **MAO inhibitors**
     amphetamine   isocarboxazid (Marplan)
     benzphetamine (Didrex)   pargyline (Eutonyl)
     dextroamphetamine   phenelzine (Nardil)
       Biphetamine, Dexedrine   tranylcypromine (Parnate)
     diethylpropion (Tenuate)
     fenfluramine (Pondimin)
     mazindol (Sanorex)
     methamphetamine (Desoxyn)
     phenmetrazine (Preludin)
     phentermine (Ionamin)

   Severity: ●●●
   Probability: ●○○

USES: Appetite suppressants are used as short-term therapy in a weight loss program. MAO inhibitors are used for some cases of clinical depression.

EFFECT: The adverse effects of the appetite suppressant may be increased. (This effect can occur for several weeks after discontinuing the MAO inhibitor.)

RESULT: Possible dangerous rise in blood pressure with symptoms such as severe headache, fever, visual disturbances, nervousness, confusion which, in severe cases, may be followed by brain hemorrhage and stroke.

WHAT TO DO: Avoid this combination.

28.   **appetite suppressants**   **urinary acidifiers**
       amphetamine   ammonium chloride
       benzphetamine (Didrex)   Ipsatol Expectorant Syrup
       dextroamphetamine   P-V-Tussin Syrup
         Biphetamine, Dexedrine   Quelldrine Syrup
       diethylpropion (Tenuate)   potassium acid phosphate
       fenfluramine (Pondimin)   K-Phos
       mazindol (Sanorex)   K-Phos No. 2
       methamphetamine (Desoxyn)   Thiacide
       phenmetrazine (Preludin)   sodium acid phosphate
       phentermine (Ionamin)   K-Phos No. 2
                                            Uroqid-Acid
                                            Uroqid-Acid No. 2

Severity: ●○○
Probability: ●●●

USES: Appetite suppressants are used as short-term therapy in a weight loss program. Urinary acidifiers: ammonium chloride is an expectorant (agent which liquefies mucus) and is used in some cough syrups; potassium acid phosphate and sodium acid phosphate are used to make the urine more acidic.

RESULT: The length of time the appetite suppressant stays in the body is decreased.

WHAT TO DO: No action appears necessary. This is an example of a "good" interaction when it is deliberately exploited in cases of amphetamine poisoning.

29. **appetite suppressants**   **urinary alkalinizers**
    amphetamine   potassium citrate
    benzphetamine (Didrex)   Alka-Seltzer
    dextroamphetamine   K-Lyte
      Biphetamine, Dexedrine   sodium acetate
    diethylpropion (Tenuate)   sodium bicarbonate
    fenfluramine (Pondimin)   Alka-Seltzer
    mazindol (Sanorex)   Citrocarbonate
    methamphetamine (Desoxyn)   sodium citrate
    phenmetrazine (Preludin)   Alka-Seltzer
    phentermine (Ionamin)   sodium lactate
                                      tromethamine

Severity: ●●○
Probability: ●●●

USES: Appetite suppressants are used as short-term therapy in a weight loss program. Urinary alkalinizers are used in some antacids and in some potassium supplement products.

EFFECT: The length of time the appetite suppressant stays in the body is increased.

RESULT: In an overdose situation, the adverse effects of the appetite suppressant will be prolonged.

WHAT TO DO: Avoid this combination.

30. ↑ **barbiturates**   **valproic acid**
    phenobarbital   **(Depakene)**
    primidone (Mysoline)

     Severity: ●●○
Probability: ●●●

USES: Phenobarbital and primidone are used for seizure disorders such as epilepsy. Valproic acid is also used for seizure disorders.

EFFECT: The effect of the barbiturate may be increased.

RESULT: Increased risk of adverse effects such as drowsiness, dizziness, loss of muscle coordination and alertness.

WHAT TO DO: Monitor the barbiturate blood level and lower the dose of the barbiturate as needed.

31. ↑ **benzodiazepines**   **birth control pills**
    alprazolam (Xanax)   Brevicon, Demulen, Genora
    chlordiazepoxide (Librium)   Levlen, Lo-Ovral, Loestrin
    clonazepam (Klonopin)   Modicon, Nelova, Norcept
    clorazepate (Tranxene)   Nordette, Norethin, Norinyl
    diazepam (Valium)   Norlestrin, Ortho-Novum
    estazolam (ProSom)   Ovcon, Ovral, Tri-Levlen
    flurazepam (Dalmane)   Tri-Norinyl
    halazepam (Paxipam)
    midazolam (Versed)
    prazepam (Centrax)
    quazepam (Doral)
    triazolam (Halcion)

     Severity: ●○○
Probability: ●○○

USES: Benzodiazepines are used for anxiety; some are used to induce sleep. Birth control pills are used to prevent pregnancy.

EFFECT: The effect of the benzodiazepine may be increased.

RESULT: Increased risk of adverse effects such as drowsiness, loss of muscle coordination and alertness.

WHAT TO DO: Watch for symptoms and lower the benzodiazepine dose as needed. Option: use a benzodiazepine which may not interact such as lorazepam (Ativan), oxazepam (Serax), temazepam (Restoril).

32. ↑ **benzodiazepines**   **cimetidine (Tagamet)**
    alprazolam (Xanax)
    chlordiazepoxide (Librium)
    clonazepam (Klonopin)
    clorazepate (Tranxene)
    diazepam (Valium)
    estazolam (ProSom)
    flurazepam (Dalmane)
    halazepam (Paxipam)
    midazolam (Versed)
    prazepam (Centrax)
    quazepam (Doral)
    triazolam (Halcion)

Severity: ●○○
Probability: ●●○

USES: Benzodiazepines are used for anxiety; some are used to induce sleep. Cimetidine is used for duodenal and gastric ulcers.

EFFECT: The effect of the benzodiazepine may be increased.

RESULT: Increased risk of adverse effects such as drowsiness, loss of muscle coordination and alertness.

WHAT TO DO: Watch for symptoms and lower the benzodiazepine dose as needed. Option: use a non-interacting benzodiazepine such as lorazepam (Ativan), oxazepam (Serax), or temazepam (Restoril); or a non-interacting alternative to cimetidine such as nizatidine (Axid) or famotidine (Pepcid).

33. ↑ **benzodiazepines**   **disulfiram (Antabuse)**
    alprazolam (Xanax)
    chlordiazepoxide (Librium)
    clonazepam (Klonopin)
    clorazepate (Tranxene)
    diazepam (Valium)
    estazolam (ProSom)
    flurazepam (Dalmane)
    halazepam (Paxipam)
    midazolam (Versed)
    prazepam (Centrax)
    quazepam (Doral)
    triazolam (Halcion)

Severity: ●○○
Probability: ●○○

USES: Benzodiazepines are used for anxiety; some are used to induce sleep. Disulfiram is prescribed to deter ingestion of alcoholic beverages.

EFFECT: The effect of the benzodiazepine may be increased.

RESULT: Increased risk of adverse effects such as drowsiness, loss of muscle coordination and alertness.

WHAT TO DO: Watch for symptoms and lower the benzodiazepine dose as needed. Option: use a non-interacting benzodiazepine such as lorazepam (Ativan), oxazepam (Serax), or temazepam (Restoril).

34. ↑ benzodiazepines   omeprazole (Prilosec)
       alprazolam (Xanax)
       chlordiazepoxide (Librium)
       clonazepam (Klonopin)
       clorazepate (Tranxene)
       diazepam (Valium)
       estazolam (ProSom)
       flurazepam (Dalmane)
       halazepam (Paxipam)
       midazolam (Versed)
       prazepam (Centrax)
       quazepam (Doral)
       triazolam (Halcion)

Severity: ●○○
Probability: ●○○

USES: Benzodiazepines are used for anxiety; some are used to induce sleep. Omeprazole is used for Gastroesophageal Reflux Disease (GERD), hypersecretory conditions, and may be approved for treatment of duodenal ulcers.

EFFECT: The effect of the benzodiazepine may be increased.

RESULT: Increased risk of adverse effects such as drowsiness, loss of muscle coordination and alertness.

WHAT TO DO: Watch for symptoms and lower the benzodiazepine dose as needed. Option: use a benzodiazepine which may not interact such as lorazepam (Ativan), oxazepam (Serax), temazepam (Restoril).

35. ↓ **benzodiazepines**   **ranitidine (Zantac)**
    diazepam (Valium)

Severity: ●●○
Probability: ●○○

USES: Benzodiazepines are used for anxiety; some are used to induce sleep. Ranitidine is used for stomach ulcers and Gastroesophageal Reflux Disease (GERD).

EFFECT: The effect of diazepam may be decreased. It isn't known whether other benzodiazepines interact.

RESULT: The condition treated with diazepam may not be properly controlled.

WHAT TO DO: Taking these drugs at different times may prevent this interaction.

36. ↓ **benzodiazepines**   **theophyllines**
    alprazolam (Xanax)   aminophylline
    chlordiazepoxide (Librium)   Somophyllin
    clonazepam (Klonopin)   dyphylline
    clorazepate (Tranxene)   Dilor, Lufyllin
    diazepam (Valium)   oxtriphylline
    estazolam (ProSom)   Choledyl
    flurazepam (Dalmane)   theophylline
    halazepam (Paxipam)   Aerolate, Bronkodyl
    lorazepam (Ativan)   Bronkaid, Constant-T
    midazolam (Versed)   Elixophyllin, Marax, Mudrane
    oxazepam (Serax)   Primatene, Quibron, Respbid
    prazepam (Centrax)   Slo-bid, Slo-Phylline
    quazepam (Doral)   T-PHYL, Tedral, Theo-24
    temazepam (Restoril)   Theo-Dur, Theo-Organidin
    triazolam (Halcion)   Theobid, Theolair
                            Theospan-SR, Theostat 80
                            Uniphyl

Severity: ●○○
Probability: ●○○

USES: Benzodiazepines are used for anxiety; some are used to induce sleep. Theophyllines are used for asthma and for bronchospasm associated with chronic bronchitis and emphysema.

EFFECT: The effect of the benzodiazepine may be decreased.

RESULT: The condition treated with the benzodiazepine may not be properly controlled.

WHAT TO DO: Use a higher dose of the benzodiazepine as needed.

37. ↓ **beta blockers**   **barbiturates**
     metoprolol (Lopressor)   amobarbital (Amytal)
     propranolol (Inderal)   aprobarbital (Alurate)
                                     butabarbital (Butisol)
                                     butalbital
                                     mephobarbital (Mebaral)
                                     pentobarbital (Nembutal)
                                     phenobarbital
                                     primidone (Mysoline)
                                     secobarbital (Seconal)
                                     talbutal (Lotusate)

   Severity: ●●○
Probability: ●●○

USES: Beta blockers are used for high blood pressure, angina heart pain, and irregular heart beats. Some have other uses, such as in the prevention of migraine headache and to calm the physical manifestations of "stage fright." Barbiturates are used as sedatives or sleep inducers; phenobarbital and primidone are used for seizure disorders such as epilepsy.

EFFECT: The effect of the beta blocker may be decreased.

RESULT: The condition treated with the beta blocker may not be properly controlled.

WHAT TO DO: Use a higher dose of the beta blocker as needed.

38. ↑ **beta blockers**   **cimetidine (Tagamet)**
     metoprolol (Lopressor)
     propranolol (Inderal)

   Severity: ●●○
Probability: ●●○

USES: Beta blockers are used for high blood pressure, angina heart pain, and irregular heart beats. Some have other uses, such as in the prevention of migraine headache and to calm the physical manifestations of "stage fright." Cimetidine is used for duodenal and gastric ulcers.

EFFECT: The effect of the beta blocker may be increased.

RESULT: Increase in adverse effects such as bradycardia (slow heart beat), fatigue, heart beat irregularities, asthma-like wheezing or difficulty breathing.

WHAT TO DO: Lower the dose of the beta blocker as needed.

39. ↑ **beta blockers**   ↑ **hydralazine**
                                                  (Apresoline)

    metoprolol (Lopressor)
    propranolol (Inderal)

Severity: ●●○
Probability: ●●○

USES: Beta blockers are used for high blood pressure, angina heart pain, and irregular heart beats. Some have other uses, such as in the prevention of migraine headache and to calm the physical manifestations of "stage fright." Hydralazine is used for high blood pressure.

EFFECT: The effect of both drugs may be increased.

RESULT: This is a "good" interaction in the sense that both drugs are sometimes used together in the treatment of high blood pressure.

WHAT TO DO: Close monitoring and adjustment of dosages may be necessary.

40. ↓ **beta blockers**   **NSAIDs**
    acebutolol (Sectral)   ibuprofen (Motrin, Rufen
    atenolol (Tenormin)   Advil, Haltran, Medipren
    betaxolol (Kerlone)   Midol 200, Pamprin-IB
    carteolol (Cartrol)   Nuprin, Trendar)
    esmolol (Brevibloc)   indomethacin (Indocin)
    metoprolol (Lopressor)   piroxicam (Feldene)
    nadolol (Corgard)   sulindac (Clinoril)
    penbutolol (Levatol)
    pindolol (Visken)
    propranolol (Inderal)
    timolol (Blocadren)

Severity: ●●○
Probability: ●●○

USES: Beta blockers are used for high blood pressure, angina heart pain, and irregular heart beats. Some have other uses, such as in the prevention of migraine headache and to calm the physical manifestations of "stage fright." NSAIDs (nonsteroidal antiinflammatory drugs) are used for the pain and inflammation of arthritis and may be used for pain and fever in general.

EFFECT: The effect of the beta blocker may be decreased.

RESULT: The condition treated with the beta blocker may not be properly controlled.

WHAT TO DO: Monitor blood pressure and use a higher dose of the beta blocker as needed. Avoid this combination if feasible.

41. ↓ **beta blockers**   **penicillins**
    atenolol (Tenormin)   ampicillin
                                     Amcill, Omnipen
                                     Polycillin, Principen

    Severity: ●●○
Probability: ●○○

USES: Beta blockers are used for high blood pressure, angina heart pain, and irregular heart beats. Some have other uses, such as in the prevention of migraine headache and to calm the physical manifestations of "stage fright." Ampicillin is an antibiotic used for microbial infections.

EFFECT: The effect of atenolol may be decreased (due to impaired absorption from the stomach).

RESULT: The condition treated with atenolol may not be properly controlled.

WHAT TO DO: Monitor the blood pressure and use a higher dose of atenolol as needed. Taking these drugs at different times may prevent this interaction.

42. ↑ **beta blockers**   ↑ **phenothiazines**
    propranolol (Inderal)   chlorpromazine (Thorazine)
                                       thioridazine (Mellaril)

    Severity: ●●○
Probability: ●●○

USES: Beta blockers are used for high blood pressure, angina heart pain, and irregular heart beats. Some have other uses, such as in the prevention of migraine headache and to calm the physical manifestations of "stage fright." Phenothiazines are antipsychotic drugs used for brain disorders such as schizophrenia, paranoia, and manic-depressive disorder.

EFFECT: The effect of both drugs may be increased.

RESULT: Increased risk of adverse effects of each drug. Beta blocker adverse effects: bradycardia (slow heart beat), fatigue, heart beat irregularities, asthma-like wheezing or difficulty breathing. Phenothiazine adverse effects: drowsiness, loss of coordination, blurry vision, dry mouth, rapid heart beat, confusion.

WHAT TO DO: Lower the dose of one or both drugs as needed.

43. ↓ **beta blockers**   **rifampin**
    metoprolol (Lopressor)   Rifadin
    propranolol (Inderal)   Rifamate
                                    Rimactane
                                    Rimactane/INH

Severity: ●●○
Probability: ●●○

USES: Beta blockers are used for high blood pressure, angina heart pain, and irregular heart beats. Some have other uses, such as in the prevention of migraine headache and to calm the physical manifestations of "stage fright." Rifampin is a specialized antibiotic used for tuberculosis and may also be given to suspected meningitis carriers.

EFFECT: The effect of the beta blocker may be decreased.

RESULT: The condition treated with the beta blocker may not be properly controlled.

WHAT TO DO: Monitor the blood pressure and use a higher dose of the beta blocker as needed.

44. ↓ **beta blockers**   **salicylates**
    acebutolol (Sectral)   aspirin
    atenolol (Tenormin)   Alka Seltzer, Anacin
    betaxolol (Kerlone)   Ascriptin, Aspergum, Bayer
    carteolol (Cartrol)   Bufferin, Cama, Ecotrin
    metoprolol (Lopressor)   Empirin, Measurin
    nadolol (Corgard)   Momentum, Persistin
                                      St. Joseph

penbutolol (Levatol)   bismuth subsalicylate
pindolol (Visken)   Pepto Bismol
propranolol (Inderal)   choline salicylate (Arthropan)
timolol (Blocadren)   magnesium salicylate
                                              Doan's
                                            salsalate (Disalcid)
                                            sodium salicylate (Uracel)
                                            sodium thiosalicylate (Tusal)

Severity: ●●○
Probability: ●○○

USES: Beta blockers are used for high blood pressure, angina heart pain, and irregular heart beats. Some have other uses, such as in the prevention of migraine headache and to calm the physical manifestations of "stage fright." Salicylates are used for the pain and inflammation of arthritis and for general pain, fever, and inflammation.

EFFECT: The blood pressure-lowering effect of the beta blocker may be decreased.

RESULT: The high blood pressure may not be properly controlled.

WHAT TO DO: Monitor the blood pressure and lower the dose of the salicylate as needed.

45. ↑ **beta blockers**   **thioamines**
     metoprolol (Lopressor)   methimazole (Tapazole)
     propranolol (Inderal)   propylthiouracil (PTU)

Severity: ●●○
Probability: ●●○

USES: Beta blockers are used for high blood pressure, angina heart pain, and irregular heart beats. Some have other uses, such as in the prevention of migraine headache and to calm the physical manifestations of "stage fright." Thioamines are used for hyperthyroidism.

EFFECT: The effect of the beta blocker may be increased.

RESULT: Increased risk of adverse effects such as bradycardia (slow heart beat), fatigue, heart beat irregularities, asthma-like wheezing or difficulty breathing.

WHAT TO DO: A lower dose of the beta blocker may be necessary when a hyperthyroid patient becomes euthyroid (normal thyroid gland function).

46. ↑ **beta blockers**   ↑ **verapamil**
(Calan, Isoptin)

acebutolol (Sectral)
atenolol (Tenormin)
betaxolol (Kerlone)
carteolol (Cartrol)
esmolol (Brevibloc)
metoprolol (Lopressor)
nadolol (Corgard)
penbutolol (Levatol)
pindolol (Visken)
propranolol (Inderal)
timolol (Blocadren)

Severity: ●●●
Probability: ●●○

USES: Beta blockers are used for high blood pressure, angina heart pain, and irregular heart beats. Some have other uses, such as in the prevention of migraine headache and to calm the physical manifestations of "stage fright." Verapamil is used for high blood pressure, angina heart pain, and irregular heart beats.

EFFECT: The adverse effects of both drugs may be increased.

RESULT: This combination can cause adverse effects on the heart and may cause the blood pressure to drop too low.

WHAT TO DO: Closely monitor heart function and lower the dose of each drug as needed.

47. ↓ **birth control pills**   **barbiturates**

Brevicon, Demulen, Genora
Levlen, Lo-Ovral, Loestrin
Modicon, Nelova, Norcept
Nordette, Norethin, Norinyl
Norlestrin, Ortho-Novum
Ovcon, Ovral, Tri-Levlen
Tri-Norinyl

amobarbital (Amytal)
aprobarbital (Alurate)
butabarbital (Butisol)
butalbital
mephobarbital (Mebaral)
pentobarbital (Nembutal)
phenobarbital
primidone (Mysoline)
secobarbital (Seconal)
talbutal (Lotusate)

Severity: ●●○
Probability: ●○○

USES: Birth control pills are used to prevent pregnancy. Barbiturates are used as sedatives or sleep inducers; phenobarbital and primidone are used for seizure disorders such as epilepsy.

EFFECT: The effect of the birth control pill may be decreased.

RESULT: Approximately 25 times increased risk of pregnancy. Breakthrough bleeding is a symptom of a possible interaction.

WHAT TO DO: Use an alternate method of contraception while taking a barbiturate.

48. ↓ **birth control pills**   **griseofulvin**
     Brevicon, Demulen, Genora   Fulvicin
     Levlen, Lo-Ovral, Loestrin   Grifulvin
     Modicon, Nelova, Norcept   Grisactin
     Nordette, Norethin, Norinyl   Gris-PEG
     Norlestrin, Ortho-Novum
     Ovcon, Ovral, Tri-Levlen
     Tri-Norinyl

     Severity: ●●○
Probability: ●○○

USES: Birth control pills are used to prevent pregnancy. Griseofulvin is an antifungal agent used for ringworm infections of the skin, hair, and nails and also for certain types of bacterial infections.

EFFECT: The effect of the birth control pill may be decreased.

RESULT: Increased risk of pregnancy. Breakthrough bleeding is a symptom of a possible interaction.

WHAT TO DO: Use an alternate method of contraception while taking griseofulvin.

49. ↓ **birth control pills**   **penicillins**
     Brevicon, Demulen, Genora   amdinocillin (Coactin)
     Levlen, Lo-Ovral, Loestrin   amoxicillin (Amoxil, Polymox)
     Modicon, Nelova, Norcept   ampicillin
     Nordette, Norethin, Norinyl   Amcill, Omnipen, Polycillin
     Norlestrin, Ortho-Novum   Principen
     Ovcon, Ovral, Tri-Levlen   azlocillin (Azlin)
     Tri-Norinyl   bacampicillin (Spectrobid)
                                        carbenicillin
                                          Geopen, Geocillin
                                        cloxacillin (Tegopen)

dicloxacillin (Dynapen)
methicillin (Staphcillin)
mezlocillin (Mezlin)
nafcillin (Unipen)
oxacillin (Prostaphlin)
penicillin G (Pentids)
penicillin V
  Betapen-VK, Pen Vee K
  Veetids
piperacillin (Pipracil)
ticarcillin (Ticar)

Severity: ●●○
Probability: ●○○

USES: Birth control pills are used to prevent pregnancy. Penicillin is an antibiotic used for microbial infections.

EFFECT: The effect of the birth control pill may be decreased.

RESULT: Increased risk of pregnancy. Breakthrough bleeding is a symptom of a possible interaction.

WHAT TO DO: Use an alternate method of contraception while taking penicillin.

50. ↓ **birth control pills**
Brevicon, Demulen, Genora
Levlen, Lo-Ovral, Loestrin
Modicon, Nelova, Norcept
Nordette, Norethin, Norinyl
Norlestrin, Ortho-Novum
Ovcon, Ovral, Tri-Levlen
Tri-Norinyl

phenytoin (Dilantin)
ethotoin (Peganone)
mephenytoin (Mesantoin)

Severity: ●●○
Probability: ●○○

USES: Birth control pills are used to prevent pregnancy. Phenytoin is used for seizure disorders such as epilepsy.

EFFECT: The effect of the birth control pill may be decreased.

RESULT: Increased risk of pregnancy. Breakthrough bleeding is a symptom of a possible interaction.

WHAT TO DO: Use an alternate method of contraception while taking phenytoin.

51. ↓ **birth control pills**   **rifampin**
Brevicon, Demulen, Genora   Rifadin
Levlen, Lo-Ovral, Loestrin   Rifamate
Modicon, Nelova, Norcept   Rimactane
Nordette, Norethin, Norinyl   Rimactane/INH
Norlestrin, Ortho-Novum
Ovcon, Ovral, Tri-Levlen
Tri-Norinyl

Severity: ●●○
Probability: ●●●

USES: Birth control pills are used to prevent pregnancy. Rifampin is a specialized antibiotic used for tuberculosis and may also be given to suspected meningitis carriers.

EFFECT: The effect of the birth control pill may be decreased.

RESULT: Increased risk of pregnancy. Breakthrough bleeding is a symptom of a possible interaction.

WHAT TO DO: Use an alternate method of contraception while taking rifampin.

52. ↓ **birth control pills**   **tetracyclines**
Brevicon, Demulen, Genora   demeclocycline (Declomycin)
Levlen, Lo-Ovral, Loestrin   doxycycline
Modicon, Nelova, Norcept   Doryx, Vibramycin, Vibra-tab
Nordette, Norethin, Norinyl   methacycline (Rondomycin)
Norlestrin, Ortho-Novum   minocycline (Minocin)
Ovcon, Ovral, Tri-Levlen   oxytetracycline (Terramycin)
Tri-Norinyl   tetracycline
                                     Achromycin V, Sumycin

Severity: ●●○
Probability: ●○○

USES: Birth control pills are used to prevent pregnancy. Tetracycline is an antibiotic used for microbial infections.

EFFECT: The effect of the birth control pill may be decreased.

RESULT: Increased risk of pregnancy. Breakthrough bleeding is a symptom of a possible interaction.

WHAT TO DO: Use an alternate method of contraception while taking tetracycline.

53. **birth control pills**   **troleandomycin (Tao)**

Brevicon, Demulen, Genora
Levlen, Lo-Ovral, Loestrin
Modicon, Nelova, Norcept
Nordette, Norethin, Norinyl
Norlestrin, Ortho-Novum
Ovcon, Ovral, Tri-Levlen
Tri-Norinyl

Severity: ●●○
Probability: ●○○

USES: Birth control pills are used to prevent pregnancy. Troleandomycin is an antibiotic used for microbial infections.

RESULT: This combination can cause cholestatic jaundice. Symptoms include loss of appetite, fatigue, itching, and a yellow discoloration of the skin and eyes.

WHAT TO DO: Avoid this combination.

54. ↑ **birth control pills**   **vitamin C**
                                          (ascorbic acid)

Brevicon, Demulen, Genora
Levlen, Lo-Ovral, Loestrin
Modicon, Nelova, Norcept
Nordette, Norethin, Norinyl
Norlestrin, Ortho-Novum
Ovcon, Ovral, Tri-Levlen
Tri-Norinyl

Severity: ●○○
Probability: ●○○

USES: Birth control pills are used to prevent pregnancy. Vitamin C is one of the essential vitamins.

EFFECT: The effect of the birth control pill may be increased.

RESULT: 1) Increase in estrogen-caused side effects. 2) If vitamin C is taken intermittently, the risk of pregnancy may be increased during the time the vitamin is *not* taken due to a "rebound" effect from the lowering of the blood level of the birth control pill's hormonal ingredients. Breakthrough bleeding is a sign of a possible interaction.

WHAT TO DO: This interaction seems to occur with larger doses of vitamin C—1000 milligrams (mg) or more daily. Taking vitamin C in the 250-500 mg range may prevent this interaction.

55. ↑ **caffeine**   **birth control pills**
No-Doz   Brevicon, Demulen, Genor
Vivarin   Levlen, Lo-Ovral, Loestrin
coffee, colas, tea   Modicon, Nelova, Norcept
nonprescription cold/pain/   Nordette, Norethin, Norinyl
   menstrual discomfort   Norlestrin, Ortho-Novum
   products (read labels)   Ovcon, Ovral, Tri-Levlen
                                          Tri-Norinyl

Severity: ●○○
Probability: ●○○

USES: Caffeine is a stimulant. Birth control pills are used to prevent pregnancy.

EFFECT: The effect of caffeine may be increased.

RESULT: Increased risk of "caffeinism" with symptoms of nervousness, agitation, irritability, insomnia, headache.

WHAT TO DO: If symptoms appear, decrease caffeine intake.

56. ↑ **caffeine**   **cimetidine (Tagamet)**
No-Doz
Vivarin
coffee, colas, tea
nonprescription cold/pain/
   menstrual discomfort
   products (read labels)

Severity: ●○○
Probability: ●○○

USES: Caffeine is a stimulant. Cimetidine is used for duodenal and gastric ulcers.

EFFECT: The effect of caffeine may be increased.

RESULT: Increased risk of "caffeinism" with symptoms of nervousness, agitation, irritability, insomnia, headache.

WHAT TO DO: If symptoms appear, decrease caffeine intake.

57. ↑ **carbamazepine**   **cimetidine (Tagamet)**
      (Epitol, tegretol)

    Severity: ●●○
Probability: ●○○

USES: Carbamazepine is used for seizure disorders such as epilepsy and for certain types of neuralgia (nerve pain). Cimetidine is used for duodenal and gastric ulcers.

EFFECT: The effect of carbamazepine may be increased to toxic levels.

RESULT: Increase in adverse effects such as dizziness, drowsiness, unsteadiness, nausea, and vomiting.

WHAT TO DO: Monitor carbamazepine blood levels and watch for symptoms of toxicity. Lower the dose of carbamazepine as needed or discontinue this combination.

58. ↑ **carbamazepine**   **danazol (Danocrine)**
      (Epitol, tegretol)

    Severity: ●●○
Probability: ●○○

USES: Carbamazepine is used for seizure disorders such as epilepsy and for certain types of neuralgia (nerve pain). Danazol is used for endometriosis (abnormally positioned endometrium, the mucous membrane lining the inner surface of the uterus), fibrocystic breast disease (lumps in the breasts), and hereditary angioedema (fluid in certain areas of the body).

EFFECT: The effect of carbamazepine may be increased to toxic levels.

RESULT: Increase in adverse effects such as dizziness, drowsiness, unsteadiness, nausea, and vomiting.

WHAT TO DO: Monitor carbamazepine blood levels and watch for symptoms of toxicity. Lower the dose of carbamazepine as needed or discontinue this combination.

59. ↑ **carbamazepine**   **erythromycin**
      (Epitol, tegretol)

                                  E.E.S., E-Mycin, Ery-Tab
                                  Eryc; EryPed, Erythrocin
                                  Eryzole, Ilosone, Ilotycin
                                  Pediazole
                                  troleandomycin (Tao)

Severity: ●●●
Probability: ●●●

USES: Carbamazepine is used for seizure disorders such as epilepsy and for certain types of neuralgia (nerve pain). Erythromycin and troleandomycin are antibiotics used for microbial infections.

EFFECT: The effect of carbamazepine may be increased to toxic levels.

RESULT: Possible medical emergency.

WHAT TO DO: Monitor carbamazepine blood levels and watch for symptoms of toxicity (dizziness, drowsiness, unsteadiness, nausea, and vomiting). Lower the dose of carbamazepine as needed or discontinue this combination.

60. ↑ carbamazepine   ↑ Isoniazid
    (Epitol, tegretol)

INH, Laniazid, Nydrazid
Rifamate, Rimactane/INH

Severity: ●●○
Probability: ●○○

USES: Carbamazepine is used for seizure disorders such as epilepsy and for certain types of neuralgia (nerve pain). Isoniazid is a specialized antibiotic used for tuberculosis.

EFFECT: The adverse effects of both drugs may be increased.

RESULT: Carbamazepine adverse effects: dizziness, drowsiness, unsteadiness, nausea, and vomiting. Isoniazid adverse effects: liver toxicity.

WHAT TO DO: Monitor carbamazepine blood levels and watch for symptoms of toxicity. Also, monitor liver function as needed. Lower the dose of carbamazepine as needed or discontinue this combination.

61. ↑ carbamazepine   propoxyphene
    (Epitol, tegretol)

Darvocet-N, Darvon, Dolene
Wygesic

Severity: ●●○
Probability: ●○○

USES: Carbamazepine is used for seizure disorders such as epilepsy and for certain types of neuralgia (nerve pain). Propoxyphene is an analgesic (pain reliever).

EFFECT: The effect of carbamazepine may be increased to toxic levels.

RESULT: Increase in adverse effects such as dizziness, drowsiness, unsteadiness, nausea, and vomiting.

WHAT TO DO: Monitor carbamazepine blood levels and watch for symptoms of toxicity. Lower the dose of carbamazepine as needed or discontinue this combination.

62. ↑ carbamazepine   verapamil
(Epitol, tegretol)   (Calan, Isoptin)

Severity: ●●○
Probability: ●○○

USES: Carbamazepine is used for seizure disorders such as epilepsy and for certain types of neuralgia (nerve pain). Verapamil is a calcium channel blocker used for high blood pressure, angina heart pain, and irregular heart beats.

EFFECT: The effect of carbamazepine may be increased to toxic levels.

RESULT: Increase in adverse effects such as dizziness, drowsiness, unsteadiness, nausea, and vomiting.

WHAT TO DO: Monitor carbamazepine blood levels and watch for symptoms of toxicity. Lower the dose (40-50% less) of carbamazepine as needed or discontinue this combination.

63. ↑ chloroquine (Aralen)   cimetidine (Tagamet)

Severity: ●○○
Probability: ●○○

USES: Chloroquine is used for malaria and extraintestinal amebiasis (infection with amebae, one-celled organisms). Cimetidine is used for duodenal and gastric ulcers.

EFFECT: The effect of chloroquine may be increased.

RESULT: Increase in adverse effects with breathing difficulties, low blood pressure and shock.

WHAT TO DO: Lower the chloroquine dose as needed.

64. ↓ **chloroquine (Aralen)**   ↓ **magnesium**
antacids (various)
milk of magnesia

Severity: ●○○
Probability: ●○○

USES: Chloroquine is used for malaria and extraintestinal amebiasis (infection with amebae, one-celled organisms). Milk of magnesia is used as a laxative.
EFFECT: Each drug may decrease the effect of the other.
RESULT: The condition treated may not be properly controlled.
WHAT TO DO: Take the two drugs 3-4 hours apart and/or use a higher dose of chloroquine.

65. ↓ **cimetidine (Tagamet)**   **antacids**
AlternaGEL, Amphojel
Camalox,Chooz, Delcid
Di-Gel, Gaviscon, Gelusil
Kudrox, Maalox, Mylanta
Riopan, Rolaids, Titralac
Tums

Severity: ●○○
Probability: ●○○

USES: Cimetidine is used for duodenal and gastric ulcers. Antacids are used for stomach problems associated with too much stomach acid.
EFFECT: The effect of cimetidine may be decreased.
RESULT: The condition treated with cimetidine may not be properly controlled.
WHAT TO DO: Take the two medications at least an hour apart if possible.

66. ↓ **clonidine**   **antidepressants, tricyclic**
Catapres   amitriptyline (Elavil, Endep)
Combipres   amoxapine (Asendin)
clomipramine (Anafranil)
desipramine
Norpramin, Pertofrane
doxepin (Adapin, Sinequan)

imipramine (Tofranil)
nortriptyline
 Aventyl, Pamelor
protriptyline (Vivactil)
trimipramine (Surmontil)

Severity: ●●●
Probability: ●●○

USES: Clonidine is used for high blood pressure. Tricyclic antidepressants are used for clinical depression.

EFFECT: The effect of clonidine may be decreased.

RESULT: Loss of blood pressure control with possibly dangerous rises in blood pressure.

WHAT TO DO: Avoid this combination if possible.

67.　**clonidine**
　　Catapres
　　Combipres

beta blockers
acebutolol (Sectral)
atenolol (Tenormin)
betaxolol (Kerlone)
carteolol (Cartrol)
esmolol (Brevibloc)
metoprolol (Lopressor)
nadolol (Corgard)
penbutolol (Levatol)
pindolol (Visken)
propranolol (Inderal)
timolol (Blocadren)

Severity: ●●●
Probability: ●○○

USES: Clonidine is used for high blood pressure. Beta blockers are used for high blood pressure, angina heart pain, and irregular heart beats; some have other uses such as for migraine headache and to calm the physical manifestations of "stage fright."

RESULT: Blood pressure control may be lost with possibly dangerous and fatal rises in blood pressure.

WHAT TO DO: Closely monitor the blood pressure. If one drug is stopped, it should be stopped gradually; it may be best to stop clonidine first.

68. ↓ **corticosteroids**

betamethasone (Celestone)
cortisone (Cortone)
dexamethasone (Decadron)
fludrocortisone (Florinef)
hydrocortisone (Cortef)
methylprednisolone (Medrol)
prednisolone (Delta-Cortef)
prednisone (Deltasone, Orasone)
triamcinolone (Aristocort)

barbiturates

amobarbital (Amytal)
aprobarbital (Alurate)
butabarbital (Butisol)
butalbital
mephobarbital (Mebaral)
pentobarbital (Nembutal)
phenobarbital
primidone (Mysoline)
secobarbital (Seconal)
talbutal (Lotusate)

Severity: ●●○
Probability: ●●●

USES: Corticosteroids are used for a wide spectrum of conditions, including arthritis, allergies, and asthma. Barbiturates are used as sedatives or as sleep inducers; phenobarbital and primidone are used for seizure disorders such as epilepsy.

EFFECT: The effect of the corticosteroid may be decreased.

RESULT: The condition treated with the corticosteroid may not be properly controlled.

WHAT TO DO: Closely monitor clinical response and use a higher dose of corticosteroid as needed. Avoid this combination if possible.

69. ↑ **corticosteroids**

hydrocortisone (Cortef)
prednisolone (Delta-Cortef)
prednisone (Deltasone, Orasone)

birth control pills

Brevicon, Demulen, Genora
Levlen, Lo-Ovral, Loestrin
Modicon, Nelova, Norcept
Nordette, Norethin, Norinyl
Norlestrin, Ortho-Novum
Ovcon, Ovral, Tri-Levlen
Tri-Norinyl

Severity: ●●○
Probability: ●○○

USES: Corticosteroids are used for a wide spectrum of conditions, including arthritis, allergies, and asthma. Birth control pills are used to prevent pregnancy.

EFFECT: The effect of certain corticosteroids may be increased.

RESULT: Increased risk of adverse effects such as high blood pressure, high blood sugar, stomach bleeding, anxiety or stimulation, depression.

WHAT TO DO: Monitor clinical response and symptoms, and lower the dose of the corticosteroid as needed.

70. ↓ **corticosteroids**   **cholestyramine**
                                          (Questran)
    hydrocortisone (Cortef)

     Severity: ●●○
    Probability: ●○○

USES: Hydrocortisone is used for a wide spectrum of conditions, including arthritis, allergies, and asthma. Cholestyramine is used to lower cholesterol blood levels.

EFFECT: The effect of hydrocortisone may be decreased.

RESULT: The condition treated with hydrocortisone may not be properly controlled.

WHAT TO DO: Use a higher dose of hydrocortisone as needed. Taking these medications several hours apart may help minimize this interaction.

71. ↑ **corticosteroids**   **erythromycin**
    methylprednisolone (Medrol)   E.E.S., E-Mycin, Ery-Tab
                                       Eryc, EryPed, Erythrocin
                                       Eryzole, Ilosone, Ilotycin
                                       Pediazole

     Severity: ●●○
    Probability: ●○○

USES: Methylprednisolone is used for a wide spectrum of conditions, including arthritis, allergies, and asthma. Erythromycin is an antibiotic used for microbial infections.

EFFECT: The effect of methylprednisolone may be increased.

RESULT: Increased risk of adverse effects such as high blood pressure, high blood sugar, stomach bleeding, anxiety or stimulation, depression.

WHAT TO DO: Closely monitor clinical response and symptoms, and lower the dose of methylprednisolone as needed.

72. ↑ **corticosteroids**
    hydrocortisone (Cortef)
    prednisolone (Delta-Cortef)
    prednisone (Deltasone,
        Orasone)

estrogens
chlorotrianisene (Tace)
conjugated estrogens
    Premarin
diethylstilbestrol (DES)
esterified estrogens
    Estratab, Menest
estradiol (Estrace)
estropipate (Ogen)
ethinyl estradiol
    Estinyl, Feminone
mestranol (Enovid)
quinestrol (Estrovis)

Severity: ●●○
Probability: ●○○

USES: Corticosteroids are used for a wide spectrum of conditions, including arthritis, allergies, and asthma. Estrogens are used for the symptoms of menopause and for osteoporosis, and also have other uses.

EFFECT: The effect of certain corticosteroids may be increased.

RESULT: Increased risk of adverse effects such as high blood pressure, high blood sugar, stomach bleeding, anxiety or stimulation, depression.

WHAT TO DO: Closely monitor clinical response and symptoms, and lower the dose of the corticosteroid as needed.

73. ↑ **corticosteroids**
    methylprednisolone (Medrol)
    prednisolone (Delta-Cortef)
    prednisone (Deltasone,
        Orasone)

ketoconazole (Nizoral)

Severity: ●●○
Probability: ●○○

USES: Corticosteroids are used for a wide spectrum of conditions, including arthritis, allergies, and asthma. Ketoconazole is used for systemic fungal infections such as thrush and for fungal infections of the skin or nails.

EFFECT: The effect of certain corticosteroids may be increased.

RESULT: Increased risk of adverse effects such as high blood pressure, high blood sugar, stomach bleeding, anxiety or stimulation, depression.

WHAT TO DO: Closely monitor clinical response and symptoms, and lower the dose of the corticosteroid as needed. Avoid this combination if possible.

74. ↓ **corticosteroids**
betamethasone (Celestone)
cortisone (Cortone)
dexamethasone (Decadron)
fludrocortisone (Florinef)
hydrocortisone (Cortef)
methylprednisolone (Medrol)
prednisolone (Delta-Cortef)
prednisone (Deltasone,
    Orasone)
triamcinolone (Aristocort)

phenytoin (Dilantin)
ethotoin (Peganone)
mephenytoin (Mesantoin)

Severity: ●●○
Probability: ●●●

USES: Corticosteroids are used for a wide spectrum of conditions, including arthritis, allergies, and asthma. Phenytoin is an anticonvulsant used for seizure disorders such as epilepsy.

EFFECT: The effect of the corticosteroid may be decreased.

RESULT: The condition treated with the corticosteroid may not be properly controlled.

WHAT TO DO: Use a higher dose (twofold or more) of the corticosteroid as needed. Avoid this combination if possible.

75. ↓ **corticosteroids**
betamethasone (Celestone)
cortisone (Cortone)
dexamethasone (Decadron)
fludrocortisone (Florinef)
hydrocortisone (Cortef)
methylprednisolone (Medrol)
prednisolone (Delta-Cortef)
prednisone (Deltasone,
    Orasone)
triamcinolone (Aristocort)

rifampin
Rifadin
Rifamate
Rimactane
Rimactane/INH

Severity: ●●○
Probability: ●●●

USES: Corticosteroids are used for a wide spectrum of conditions, including arthritis, allergies, and asthma. Rifampin is a specialized antibiotic used for tuberculosis and may also be given to suspected meningitis carriers.

EFFECT: The effect of the corticosteroid may be decreased.

RESULT: The condition treated with the corticosteroid may not be properly controlled.

WHAT TO DO: Use a higher dose (twofold or more) of the corticosteroid as needed. Avoid this combination if possible.

76. ↑ **corticosteroids**   **troleandomycin (Tao)**
      methylprednisolone
         (Medrol)

Severity: ●●○
Probability: ●●●

USES: Corticosteroids are used for a wide spectrum of conditions, including arthritis, allergies, and asthma. Troleandomycin is an antibiotic used for microbial infections.

EFFECT: The effect of methylprednisolone may be increased. (It is not certain whether other corticosteroids interact this way.)

RESULT: Increased risk of adverse effects such as high blood pressure, high blood sugar, stomach bleeding, anxiety or stimulation, depression.

WHAT TO DO: Closely monitor clinical response and symptoms, and lower the dose of the corticosteroid as needed. (This has been used as a "good interaction" since it makes possible a lower dose of methylprednisolone in corticosteroid-treated asthmatics.)

77. ↑ **cyclosporine**   **diltiazem (Cardizem)**
         (Sandimmune)

Severity: ●●○
Probability: ●○○

USES: Cyclosporine is an immunosuppressant used to prevent rejection of a transplanted organ. Diltiazem is a beta blocker drug used for high blood pressure, angina heart pain, and irregular heart beats.

EFFECT: The effect of cyclosporine may be increased.

RESULT: Increased suppression of the immune system and possibly kidney toxicity.

WHAT TO DO: Closely monitor cyclosporine blood levels and serum creatinine. Lower the dose of cyclosporine or use an alternative to diltiazem as needed.

78. **↑ cyclosporine**   **erythromycin**
      (Sandimmune)

> E.E.S., E-Mycin, Ery-Tab
> Eryc, EryPed, Erythrocin
> Eryzole, Ilosone, Ilotycin
> Pediazole

Severity: ●●○
Probability: ●●●

USES: Cyclosporine is an immunosuppressant used to prevent rejection of a transplanted organ. Erythromycin is an antibiotic used for microbial infections.

EFFECT: The effect of cyclosporine may be increased.

RESULT: Increased suppression of the immune system and possibly kidney toxicity.

WHAT TO DO: Closely monitor cyclosporine blood levels and serum creatinine. Lower the dose of cyclosporine as needed.

79. **↑ cyclosporine**   **ketoconazole (Nizoral)**
      (Sandimmune)

Severity: ●●○
Probability: ●○○

USES: Cyclosporine is an immunosuppressant used to prevent rejection of a transplanted organ. Ketoconazole is used for systemic fungal infections such as thrush and for fungal infections of the skin or nails.

EFFECT: The effect of cyclosporine may be increased. This effect may persist for a week or more after this combination is stopped.

RESULT: Increased suppression of the immune system and possibly kidney toxicity.

WHAT TO DO: Closely monitor cyclosporine blood levels and serum creatinine. Lower the dose of cyclosporine as needed.

80. ↑ **cyclosporine**   **metoclopramide**
       (Sandimmune)   **(Reglan)**

    Severity: ●●○
Probability: ●○○

USES: Cyclosporine is an immunosuppressant used to prevent rejection of a transplanted organ. Metoclopramide is used for gastroesophageal reflux disease (GERD) and for nausea and vomiting associated with certain types of cancer chemotherapy.

EFFECT: The effect of cyclosporine may be increased.

RESULT: Increased suppression of the immune system and possibly kidney toxicity.

WHAT TO DO: Closely monitor cyclosporine blood levels and serum creatinine. Lower the dose of cyclosporine as needed.

81. ↓ **cyclosporine**   **phenytoin (Dilantin)**
       (Sandimmune)

                                   ethotoin (Peganone)
                                   mephenytoin (Mesantoin)

    Severity: ●●●
Probability: ●●○

USES: Cyclosporine is an immunosuppressant used to prevent rejection of a transplanted organ. Phenytoin is an anticonvulsant used for seizure disorders such as epilepsy.

EFFECT: The effect of cyclosporine may be decreased. This effect appears to subside within a week of stopping phenytoin use.

RESULT: Decrease in immunosuppressant action leading to possible rejection of a transplanted organ.

WHAT TO DO: Closely monitor cyclosporine blood levels and serum creatinine. Use a higher dose of cyclosporine as needed.

82. ↓ **cyclosporine**   **rifampin**
       (Sandimmune)

                                     Rifadin
                                     Rifamate
                                     Rimactane
                                     Rimactane/INH

Severity: ●●●
Probability: ●○○

USES: Cyclosporine is an immunosuppressant used to prevent rejection of a transplanted organ. Rifampin is a specialized antibiotic used for tuberculosis and may also be given to suspected meningitis carriers.

EFFECT: The effect of cyclosporine may be decreased. This effect may persist for up to three weeks after stopping rifampin.

RESULT: Decrease in immunosuppressant action leading to possible rejection of a transplanted organ.

WHAT TO DO: Closely monitor cyclosporine blood levels and serum creatinine. Use a higher dose of cyclosporine as needed. Avoid this combination if possible.

---

83. **dextromethorphan (DM)**   **MAO Inhibitors**
numerous cough preparations   isocarboxazid (Marplan)
  e.g., Benylin DM   pargyline (Eutonyl)
  Robitussin-DM   phenelzine (Nardil)
          tranylcypromine (Parnate)

Severity: ●●●
Probability: ●○○

USES: Dextromethorphan is the cough suppressant found in numerous nonprescription cough preparations (read product labels). MAO inhibitors are used for some cases of clinical depression.

RESULT: Possible extreme fever, dangerous fall in blood pressure, coma. A death has been reported.

WHAT TO DO: Avoid this combination if possible.

---

84. ↓ **digitoxin (Crystodigin)**   **cholestyramine**
          (Questran)

Severity: ●●○
Probability: ●●○

USES: Digitoxin is used for congestive heart failure and other heart disorders. Cholestyramine is used to lower cholesterol blood levels.

EFFECT: The effect of digitoxin may be decreased.

RESULT: The condition treated with digitoxin may not be properly controlled.

WHAT TO DO: Monitor clinical response and digitoxin blood levels and use a higher dose of digitoxin as needed.

85. ↓ **digitoxin (Crystodigin)**   **colestipol (Colestid)**

Severity: ●●○
Probability: ●○○

USES: Digitoxin is used for congestive heart failure and other heart disorders. Colestipol is used to lower cholesterol blood levels.

EFFECT: The effect of digitoxin may be decreased.

RESULT: The condition treated with digitoxin may not be properly controlled.

WHAT TO DO: Monitor clinical response and digitoxin blood levels and use a higher dose of digitoxin as needed.

86. ↑ **digitoxin (Crystodigin)**   **quinidine**
Cardioquin, Cin-Quin
Duraquin, Quinaglute
Dura-Tabs, Quinalan
Quinidex, Extentabs
Quinora

Severity: ●●●
Probability: ●●○

USES: Digitoxin is used for congestive heart failure and other heart disorders. Quinidine is used for heart beat irregularities.

EFFECT: The effect of digitoxin may be significantly increased to toxic levels.

RESULT: Increased risk of adverse effects such as heart beat irregularities, loss of appetite, visual disturbances (blurred or yellow vision), nausea, vomiting, headache, weakness, dizziness, apathy.

WHAT TO DO: Monitor digitoxin blood levels and symptoms, and lower the dose of digitoxin (30-70% lower) as needed.

87. ↓ **digitoxin (Crystodigin)**   **rifampin**
Rifadin
Rifamate
Rimactane
Rimactane/INH

Severity: ●●○
Probability: ●○○

USES: Digitoxin is used for congestive heart failure and other heart disorders. Rifampin is a specialized antibiotic used for tuberculosis and may also be given to suspected meningitis carriers.

EFFECT: The effect of digitoxin may be decreased.

RESULT: The condition treated with digitoxin may not be properly controlled.

WHAT TO DO: Monitor clinical response and digitoxin blood levels and use a higher dose of digitoxin as needed.

88. ↑ **digitoxin (Crystodigin)**   **verapamil**
                                       (Calan, Isoptin)

   Severity: ●●○
Probability: ●○○

USES: Digitoxin is used for congestive heart failure and other heart disorders. Verapamil is a calcium channel blocker used for high blood pressure, angina heart pain, and irregular heart beats.

EFFECT: The effect of digitoxin may be increased to toxic levels.

RESULT: Increased risk of adverse effects such as heart beat irregularities, loss of appetite, visual disturbances (blurred or yellow vision), nausea, vomiting, headache, weakness, dizziness, apathy.

WHAT TO DO: Monitor digitoxin blood levels and symptoms, and lower the dose of digitoxin as needed.

89. ↓ **digoxin (Lanoxin)**   **aminoglycosides, oral**
                                       kanamycin (Kantrex)
                                       neomycin
                                         Mycifradin, Neobiotic
                                       paromomycin (Humatin)

   Severity: ●●○
Probability: ●○○

USES: Digoxin is used for congestive heart failure and other heart disorders. Aminoglycosides are a specialized type of antibiotic.

EFFECT: The effect of digoxin may be decreased.

RESULT: The condition treated with digoxin may not be properly controlled.

WHAT TO DO: Monitor clinical response and digoxin blood levels and use a higher dose of digoxin as needed.

90. ↑ **digoxin (Lanoxin)**   **amiodarone
                                                      (Cordarone)**

      Severity: ●●●
Probability: ●●○

USES: Digoxin is used for congestive heart failure and other heart disorders. Amiodarone is recommended only for life-threatening heart beat irregularities of the ventricular type.

EFFECT: The effect of digoxin may be increased to toxic levels.

RESULT: Increased risk of adverse effects such as heart beat irregularities, loss of appetite, visual disturbances (blurred or yellow vision), nausea, vomiting, headache, weakness, dizziness, apathy.

WHAT TO DO: Monitor digoxin blood levels and symptoms, and lower the dose of digoxin as needed.

91. ↓ **digoxin (Lanoxin)**   **antineoplastic agents**
                                                      bleomycin (Blenoxane)
                                                      carmustine (BiCNU)
                                                      cyclophosphamide
                                                        Cytoxan, Neosar
                                                      cytarabine (Cytosar-U)
                                                      doxorubicin (Adriamycin)
                                                      methotrexate (Folex, Mexate)
                                                      procarbazine (Matulane)
                                                      vincristine (Oncovin)

      Severity: ●●○
Probability: ●○○

USES: Digoxin is used for congestive heart failure and other heart disorders. Antineoplastic agents are used as chemotherapy for cancer.

EFFECT: The effect of digoxin may be decreased.

RESULT: The condition treated with digoxin may not be properly controlled.

WHAT TO DO: Monitor digoxin blood levels and clinical response, and use a higher dose of digoxin as needed. The use of Lanoxicaps (capsule form of Lanoxin) or digitoxin (Crystodigin) may minimize this interaction.

92. ↓ **digoxin (Lanoxin)**   **cholestyramine**
                                              (Questran)

Severity: ●●○
Probability: ●●○

USES: Digoxin is used for congestive heart failure and other heart disorders. Cholestyramine is used to lower cholesterol blood levels.

EFFECT: The effect of digoxin may be decreased.

RESULT: The condition treated with digoxin may not be properly controlled.

WHAT TO DO: Monitor digoxin blood levels and clinical response, and use a higher dose of digoxin as needed. Taking the medications eight hours apart appears to minimize this interaction. Also, use of digoxin capsules in place of tablets may minimize this interaction. (This can be a "good interaction" since it can be used in treating digoxin toxicity or overdose.)

93. ↓ **digoxin (Lanoxin)**   **colestipol (Colestid)**

Severity: ●●○
Probability: ●○○

USES: Digoxin is used for congestive heart failure and other heart disorders. Colestipol is used to lower cholesterol blood levels.

EFFECT: The effect of digoxin may be decreased.

RESULT: The condition treated with digoxin may not be properly controlled.

WHAT TO DO: Monitor digoxin blood levels and clinical response, and use a higher dose of digoxin as needed. Taking the medications eight hours apart may minimize this interaction. This can be a "good interaction" since it can be used in treating digoxin toxicity or overdose.

94. ↑ **digoxin (Lanoxin)**   **cyclosporine**
                                              (Sandimmune)

Severity: ●●●
Probability: ●○○

USES: Digoxin is used for congestive heart failure and other heart disorders. Cyclosporine is an immunosuppressant used to prevent rejection of a transplanted organ.

EFFECT: The effect of digoxin may be increased to toxic levels.

RESULT: Increased risk of adverse effects such as heart beat irregularities, loss of appetite, visual disturbances (blurred or yellow vision), nausea, vomiting, headache, weakness, dizziness, apathy.

WHAT TO DO: Monitor digoxin blood levels and symptoms, and lower the dose of digoxin as needed.

95. **digoxin (Lanoxin)**
digitalis (Digifortis)
digitoxin (Crystodigin)

diuretics, loop
bumetanide (Bumex)
ethacrynic acid (Edecrin)
furosemide (Lasix)

Severity: ●●●
Probability: ●●○

USES: Digoxin and the other listed preparations are used for congestive heart failure and other heart disorders. Diuretics are used to rid the body of excess fluid—this makes them effective in treating congestive heart failure, high blood pressure, cirrhosis of the liver, and kidney dysfunction.

RESULT: The loss of electrolytes (potassium and magnesium) caused by the diuretic may lead to digoxin-induced heart beat disturbances.

WHAT TO DO: Monitor blood levels of potassium and magnesium as needed. Taking a potassium/magnesium supplement may be necessary. Other options include restricting dietary sodium (sodium may facilitate the loss of potassium) and use of a different type of diuretic (called potassium-sparing) that does not cause potassium loss.

96. **digoxin (Lanoxin)**
digitalis (Digifortis)
digitoxin (Crystodigin)/

diuretics, thiazide
bendroflumethiazide
    Naturetin
benzthiazide (Aquatag)
chlorothiazide (Diuril)
chlorthalidone (Hygroton)
cyclothiazide (Anhydron)
hydrochlorothiazide
    Esidrix, HydroDiuril
hydroflumethiazide (Saluron)
indapamide (Lozol)
methyclothiazide (Enduron)

metolazone
 Diulo, Zaroxolyn
polythiazide (Renese)
quinethazone (Hydromox)
trichlormethiazide (Naqua)

Severity: ●●●
Probability: ●●○

USES: Digoxin and the other listed preparations are used for congestive heart failure and other heart disorders. Diuretics are used to rid the body of excess fluid—this makes them effective in treating congestive heart failure, high blood pressure, cirrhosis of the liver, and kidney dysfunction.

RESULT: The loss of electrolytes (potassium and magnesium) caused by the diuretic may lead to digoxin-induced heart beat disturbances.

WHAT TO DO: Monitor blood levels of potassium and magnesium as needed. Taking a potassium/magnesium supplement may be necessary. Other options include restricting dietary sodium (sodium may facilitate the loss of potassium) and use of a different type of diuretic (called potassium-sparing) that does not cause potassium loss.

97. ↑ **digoxin (Lanoxin)**

erythromycin
E.E.S., E-Mycin, Ery-Tab
Eryc, EryPed, Erythrocin
Eryzole, Ilosone, Ilotycin
Pediazole

Severity: ●●●
Probability: ●●○

USES: Digoxin is used for congestive heart failure and other heart disorders. Erythromycin is an antibiotic used for microbial infections.

EFFECT: The effect of digoxin may be increased to toxic levels. This occurs only in about 10% of individuals—those whose GI tract breaks down digoxin in a certain way. This effect can occur for several weeks after stopping erythromycin.

RESULT: Increased risk of adverse effects such as heart beat irregularities, loss of appetite, visual disturbances (blurred or yellow vision), nausea, vomiting, headache, weakness, dizziness, apathy.

WHAT TO DO: Monitor digoxin blood levels and symptoms, and lower the dose of digoxin as needed.

98. ↓ **digoxin (Lanoxin)**   **metoclopramide**
                                                          (Reglan)

     Severity: ●●○
Probability: ●●○

USES: Digoxin is used for congestive heart failure and other heart disorders. Metoclopramide is used for gastroesophageal reflux disease (GERD) and for nausea and vomiting associated with certain types of cancer chemotherapy.

EFFECT: The effect of digoxin may be decreased.

RESULT: The condition treated with digoxin may not be properly controlled.

WHAT TO DO: Monitor digoxin blood levels and clinical response, and use a higher dose of digoxin as needed. Taking a digoxin tablet with a reliably high dissolution rate—eg, Lanoxin brand tablet—rather than a generic tablet, or taking digoxin in the capsule or elixir form minimizes the potential for this interaction.

99. ↓ **digoxin (Lanoxin)**   **penicillamine**
                                                          Cuprimine
                                                          Depen

     Severity: ●●○
Probability: ●○○

USES: Digoxin is used for congestive heart failure and other heart disorders. Penicillamine is used for Wilson's disease (a genetic disorder causing an abnormality in copper metabolism), cystinuria (amino acids in the urine), and severe rheumatoid arthritis.

EFFECT: The effect of digoxin may be decreased.

RESULT: The condition treated with digoxin may not be properly controlled.

WHAT TO DO: Monitor digoxin blood levels and clinical response, and use a higher dose of digoxin as needed.

100. ↓ **digoxin (Lanoxin)**   **phenytoin (Dilantin)**
          digitoxin (Crystodigin)   ethotoin (Peganone)
                                                          mephenytoin (Mesantoin)

     Severity: ●●○
Probability: ●○○

USES: Digoxin is used for congestive heart failure and other heart disorders. Phenytoin is an anticonvulsant used for seizure disorders such as epilepsy.

EFFECT: The effect of digoxin may be decreased.

RESULT: The condition treated with digoxin may not be properly controlled.

WHAT TO DO: Monitor digoxin blood levels and clinical response, and use a higher dose of digoxin as needed.

101. ↑digoxin (Lanoxin)

quinidine
Cardioquin, Cin-Quin
Duraquin, Quinaglute
Dura-Tabs, Quinalan
Quinidex, Extentabs
Quinora

Severity: ●●●
Probability: ●●●

USES: Digoxin is used for congestive heart failure and other heart disorders. Quinidine is used for heart beat irregularities.

EFFECT: The effect of digoxin may be increased to toxic levels.

RESULT: Increase in adverse effects of digoxin with symptoms such as heart beat irregularities, nausea, vomiting, loss of appetite, headache, weakness, dizziness, and blurred or yellow vision.

WHAT TO DO: Closely monitor digoxin blood levels and symptoms, and lower the dose of digoxin (50% less when quinidine is started) as needed.

102. ↑digoxin (Lanoxin)

quinine
Quin-260
Quinamm
Quine
Quinite

Severity: ●●○
Probability: ●●○

USES: Digoxin is used for congestive heart failure and other heart disorders. Quinine is used for nighttime leg muscle cramps. It is available over-the-counter in various brand names.

EFFECT: The effect of digoxin may be increased to toxic levels.

RESULT: Increased risk of adverse effects such as heart beat irregularities, loss of appetite, visual disturbances (blurred or yellow vision), nausea, vomiting, headache, weakness, dizziness, apathy.

WHAT TO DO: Closely monitor digoxin blood levels and symptoms, and lower the dose of digoxin as needed.

103. ↑ digoxin (Lanoxin)   **tetracyclines**

demeclocycline (Declomycin)
doxycycline
  Doryx, Vibramycin, Vibra-tab
methacycline (Rondomycin)
minocycline (Minocin)
oxytetracycline (Terramycin)
tetracycline
  Achromycin V, Sumycin

Severity: ●●●
Probability: ●○○

USES: Digoxin is used for congestive heart failure and other heart disorders. Tetracycline is an antibiotic used for microbial infections.

EFFECT: The effect of digoxin may be increased to toxic levels. This occurs only in about 10% of individuals—those whose GI tract breaks down digoxin in a certain way. This effect can occur for several weeks or months after stopping tetracycline.

RESULT: Increased risk of adverse effects such as heart beat irregularities, loss of appetite, visual disturbances (blurred or yellow vision), nausea, vomiting, headache, weakness, dizziness, apathy.

WHAT TO DO: Closely monitor digoxin blood levels and symptoms, and lower the dose of digoxin as needed.

104. ↑ digoxin (Lanoxin)   **thioamines**
digitalis (Digifortis)   methimazole (Tapazole)
digitoxin (Crystodigin)   propylthiouracil (PTU)

Severity: ●●○
Probability: ●●●

USES: Digoxin and the other listed preparations are used for congestive heart failure and other heart disorders. Thioamines are antithyroid agents used for hyperthyroidism.

EFFECT: The effect of digoxin may be increased to toxic levels.

RESULT: Increased risk of adverse effects such as heart beat irregularities, loss of appetite, visual disturbances (blurred or yellow vision), nausea, vomiting, headache, weakness, dizziness, apathy.

WHAT TO DO: Patients currently maintained on thioamines who are started on digoxin require no special monitoring. However, patients currently taking digoxin who subsequently require thioamine treatment may require a lower dose of digoxin. Monitor digoxin blood levels and symptoms and lower the digoxin dose as needed.

105. ↓ digoxin (Lanoxin)   thyroid
digitalis (Digifortis)   dextrothyroxine (Choloxin)
digitoxin (Crystodigin)   levothyroxine (Synthroid)
                                liothyronine (Cytomel)
                                 liotrix (Euthroid, Thyrolar)
                                thyroglobulin (Proloid)
                                thyroid (Armour thyroid)

Severity: ●●○
Probability: ●●●

USES: Digoxin and the other listed preparations are used for congestive heart failure and other heart disorders. Thyroid is used for hypothyroidism and for goiters (enlargements of the thyroid gland).

EFFECT: The effect of digoxin may be decreased.

RESULT: The condition treated by digoxin may not be properly controlled.

WHAT TO DO: Patients currently maintained on thyroid who are started on digoxin require no special monitoring. However, patients currently taking digoxin who subsequently require thyroid treatment may require a higher dose of digoxin. Monitor digoxin blood levels and clinical response, and use a higher digoxin dose as needed.

106. ↑ digoxin (Lanoxin)   verapamil
                                (Calan, Isoptin)

Severity: ●●●
Probability: ●●●

USES: Digoxin is used for congestive heart failure and other heart disorders. Verapamil is a calcium channel blocker used for high blood pressure, angina heart pain, and irregular heart beats.

EFFECT: The effect of digoxin may be increased to toxic levels.

RESULT: Increased risk of adverse effects such as heart beat irregularities, loss of appetite, visual disturbances (blurred or yellow vision), nausea, vomiting, headache, weakness, dizziness, apathy.

WHAT TO DO: Closely monitor digoxin blood levels and symptoms, and lower the dose of digoxin as needed.

---

107.   ↓disopyramide (Norpace)   phenytoin (Dilantin)
                                        ethotoin (Peganone)
                                        mephenytoin (Mesantoin)

      Severity: ●●○
Probability: ●○○

USES: Disopyramide is used for heart beat irregularities. Phenytoin is an anticonvulsant used for seizure disorders such as epilepsy.

EFFECT: The effect of disopyramide may be decreased.

RESULT: The condition treated with disopyramide may not be properly controlled. In addition, anticholinergic side effects (dry mouth, blurred vision, dizziness, constipation, difficult urination) may increase due to a breakdown product of disopyramide.

WHAT TO DO: Use a higher dose of disopyramide as needed. If anticholinergic side effects become significant, use of an alternative to disopyramide may be necessary.

---

108.   disulfiram (Antabuse)   metronidazole
                                        Flagyl, Metryl, Protostat

      Severity: ●●○
Probability: ●○○

USES: Disulfiram is prescribed to deter ingestion of alcoholic beverages. Metronidazole is used for trichomoniasis, a type of vaginitis, and for acute amoebic dysentery.

RESULT: This combination may cause confusion, aberrant or psychotic behavior.

WHAT TO DO: If adverse symptoms develop, stop one or both drugs. Avoid this combination if possible.

109. ↓ **diuretics, loop**   **NSAIDs**
  bumetanide (Bumex)   ibuprofen (Motrin, Rufen
  ethacrynic acid (Edecrin)   Advil, Haltran, Medipren
  furosemide (Lasix)   Midol 200, Pamprin-IB
                                               Nuprin, Trendar)
                                              indomethacin (Indocin)
                                              sulindac (Clinoril)

  Severity: ●○○
Probability: ●●○

USES: Diuretics are used to rid the body of excess fluid—this makes them effective in treating congestive heart failure, high blood pressure, cirrhosis of the liver, and kidney dysfunction. NSAIDs (nonsteroidal antiinflammatory drugs) are used for pain and inflammation in arthritic-type conditions and for general pain and inflammation.

EFFECT: The effect of the diuretic may be decreased.

RESULT: The condition treated with the diuretic may not be properly controlled.

WHAT TO DO: Use a higher dose of the diuretic as needed. An option is to use another NSAID such as flurbiprofen (Ansaid).

110. ↓ **diuretics, loop**   **phenytoin (Dilantin)**
  furosemide (Lasix)   ethotoin (Peganone)
                                              mephenytoin (Mesantoin)

  Severity: ●○○
Probability: ●○○

USES: Furosemide is a diuretic used to rid the body of excess fluid, which makes it effective in treating congestive heart failure, high blood pressure, cirrhosis of the liver, and kidney dysfunction. Phenytoin is an anticonvulsant used for seizure disorders such as epilepsy.

EFFECT: The effect of furosemide may be decreased.

RESULT: The condition treated with furosemide may not be properly controlled.

WHAT TO DO: Use a higher dose of furosemide as needed.

111. ↓ **diuretics, thiazide**   **cholestyramine**
                                              (Questran)

    bendroflumethiazide
     Naturetin
    benzthiazide (Aquatag)
    chlorothiazide (Diuril)
    chlorthalidone (Hygroton)
    cyclothiazide (Anhydron)
    hydrochlorothiazide
     Esidrix, HydroDiuril
    hydroflumethiazide (Saluron)
    indapamide (Lozol)
    methyclothiazide (Enduron)
    metolazone
     Diulo, Zaroxolyn
    polythiazide (Renese)
    quinethazone (Hydromox)
    trichlormethiazide (Naqua)

  Severity: ●○○
Probability: ●●○

USES: Diuretics are used to rid the body of excess fluid—this makes them effective in treating congestive heart failure, high blood pressure, cirrhosis of the liver, and kidney dysfunction. Cholestyramine is used to lower blood cholesterol levels.

EFFECT: The effect of the diuretic may be decreased.

RESULT: The condition treated with the diuretic may not be properly controlled.

WHAT TO DO: Take the two medications two hours or more apart. A higher dose of the diuretic may still be necessary.

112. ↓ **diuretics, thiazide**   **colestipol (Colestid)**
    bendroflumethiazide
     Naturetin
    benzthiazide (Aquatag)
    chlorothiazide (Diuril)
    chlorthalidone (Hygroton)
    cyclothiazide (Anhydron)
    hydrochlorothiazide
     Esidrix, HydroDiuril
    hydroflumethiazide (Saluron)
    indapamide (Lozol)

methyclothiazide (Enduron)
metolazone (Diulo,
    Zaroxolyn)
polythiazide (Renese)
quinethazone (Hydromox)
trichlormethiazide (Naqua)

Severity: ●○○
Probability: ●○○

USES: Diuretics are used to rid the body of excess fluid—this makes them effective in treating congestive heart failure, high blood pressure, cirrhosis of the liver, and kidney dysfunction. Colestipol is used to lower blood cholesterol levels.

EFFECT: The effect of the diuretic may be decreased.

RESULT: The condition treated with the diuretic may not be properly controlled.

WHAT TO DO: Take the two medications two hours or more apart. A higher dose of the diuretic may still be necessary.

113. ↓ **doxycycline**
    Doryx
    Vibramycin
    Vibra-Tabs

barbiturates
amobarbital (Amytal)
aprobarbital (Alurate)
butabarbital (Butisol)
butalbital
mephobarbital (Mebaral)
pentobarbital (Nembutal)
phenobarbital
primidone (Mysoline)
secobarbital (Seconal)
talbutal (Lotusate)

Severity: ●●○
Probability: ●○○

USES: Doxycycline is an antibiotic used for microbial infections. Barbiturates are used as sedatives or sleep inducers; phenobarbital and primidone are used for seizure disorders such as epilepsy.

EFFECT: The effect of doxycycline may be decreased.

RESULT: The infection treated with doxycycline may not be properly controlled.

WHAT TO DO: Use a higher dose of doxycycline as needed. Option: use an alternative to doxycycline.

114. ↓ **doxycycline**   **carbamazepine**
                                              (Epitol, Tegretol)

    Doryx
    Vibramycin
    Vibra-Tabs

    Severity: ●●○
Probability: ●○○

USES: Doxycycline is an antibiotic used for microbial infections.
Carbamazepine is used for seizure disorders such as epilepsy and
for trigeminal neuralgia (severe pain in a facial nerve), also known
as *tic douloureux.*

EFFECT: The effect of doxycycline may be decreased.

RESULT: The infection treated with doxycycline may not be properly
controlled.

WHAT TO DO: Use a higher dose of doxycycline as needed. Option:
use an alternative to doxycycline.

115. ↓ **doxycycline**   **phenytoin (Dilantin)**
    Doryx   ethotoin (Peganone)
    Vibramycin   mephenytoin (Mesantoin)
    Vibra-Tabs

    Severity: ●●○
Probability: ●●○

USES: Doxycycline is an antibiotic used for microbial infections.
Phenytoin is an anticonvulsant used for seizure disorders such as
epilepsy.

EFFECT: The effect of doxycycline may be significantly decreased.

RESULT: The infection treated with doxycycline may not be properly
controlled.

WHAT TO DO: Use a higher dose of doxycycline as needed. Option:
use an alternative to doxycycline.

116. ↑ **dyphylline**   **probenecid**
       (Dilor, Lufyllin)

                                              Benemid
                                              ColBenemid

    Severity: ●●○
Probability: ●●○

USES: Dyphylline is used for asthma and for bronchospasm associated with chronic bronchitis and emphysema. Probenecid is used for gout and gouty arthritis.

EFFECT: The effect of dyphylline may be increased.

RESULT: Increased risk of adverse effects such as tremors, rapid heart beat, heart beat irregularities, nausea, dizziness, headache, irritability.

WHAT TO DO: Watch for symptoms and lower the dose of dyphylline as needed. Option: use an alternative to dyphylline such as theophylline, which does not appear to interact with probenecid.

117. **ergots** **beta blockers**

ergotamine carteolol (Cartrol)
  Bellergal-S nadolol (Corgard)
  Cafergot penbutolol (Levatol)
  Ergomar pindolol (Visken)
  Ergostat propranolol (Inderal)
  Wigraine timolol (Blocadren)
methysergide (Sansert)

Severity: ●●○
Probability: ●○○

USES: Ergot preparations are used for vascular or migraine headache. Beta blockers are used for high blood pressure, angina heart pain, and irregular heart beats; some have other uses such as for migraine headache and to calm the physical manifestations of "stage fright."

EFFECT: Ischemia (obstruction of blood flow) to the outer body parts.

RESULT: Extremities may feel cold, and gangrene (tissue death) is a possibility.

WHAT TO DO: Monitor for signs of the problem. Adjust the ergot dose or stop the beta blocker as needed.

118. ↓ **erythromycin** **food**
Erythrocin
erythromycin in capsule
    form
erythromycin uncoated
    tablet

Severity: ●●○
Probability: ●○○

USES: Erythromycin is an antibiotic used for microbial infections.

EFFECT: The effect of erythromycin may be decreased. This occurs with erythromycin in stearate form (Erythrocin), in capsule form, and in non-enteric coated tablets.

RESULT: The infection treated with erythromycin may not be properly controlled.

WHAT TO DO: Take the above listed forms of erythromcyin two hours before or after meals. The following erythromycin products may be given without regard to meals: E.E.S., E-Mycin, Ery-Tab, Eryc, EryPed, Eryzole, Ilosone, Ilotycin, Pediazole.

119. ↓ folic acid   sulfasalazine
                                              (Azulfidine)

   Severity: ●○○
Probability: ●○○

USES: Folic acid is an essential vitamin found in liver, yeast, green leafy vegetables, and fruits, and in some vitamin supplements. Sulfasalazine is used for ulcerative colitis.

EFFECT: Possible loss of folic acid from the body.

RESULT: Folic acid deficiency may occur.

WHAT TO DO: Increase dietary folic acid, take sulfasalazine between meals, or take a folic acid supplement (e.g., Folvite) as needed.

120.   food, amine-containing   furazolidone
                                         (Furoxone)

        avocados, baked potatoes
        bananas, bean pods, beer
        bologna, Brie, broad beans
        caviar, cheeses, chicken liver
        figs (canned), meat
        tenderizers, nuts, packet
        soups, pepperoni, pickled
        herring, raspberries, salami
        sauerkraut, summer sausage
        sour cream, soy sauce, wines
        yeast, yogurt

   Severity: ●●●
Probability: ●●●

USES: Furazolidone is used for bacterial and protozoal diarrhea and enteritis (inflammation of the intestines).

EFFECT: Possible dangerous rise in blood pressure. (This effect can occur even several weeks after furazolidone is discontinued.)

RESULT: Symptoms include severe headache, fever, visual disturbances, and confusion which may be followed by brain hemorrhage/stroke.

WHAT TO DO: Avoid amine-containing foods.

121. **food, amine-containing**
avocados, baked potatoes, bananas, bean pods, beer, bologna, Brie, broad beans, caviar, cheeses, chicken liver, figs (canned), meat tenderizers, nuts, packet soups, pepperoni, pickled herring, raspberries, salami, sauerkraut, summer sausage, sour cream, soy sauce, wines, yeast, yogurt

MAO inhibitors
isocarboxazid (Marplan)
pargyline (Eutonyl)
phenelzine (Nardil)
tranylcypromine (Parnate)

Severity: ●●●
Probability: ●●●

USES: MAO inhibitors are used for some cases of clinical depression.

EFFECT: Possible dangerous rise in blood pressure. (This effect can occur even several weeks after the MAO inhibitor is discontinued.)

RESULT: Severe headache, fever, visual disturbances, confusion which may be followed by brain hemorrhage/stroke.

WHAT TO DO: Avoid amine-containing foods.

122. ↓ **griseofulvin**
Fulvicin
Grifulvin V
Grisactin
Gris-PEG

barbiturates
amobarbital (Amytal)
aprobarbital (Alurate)
butalbital
butabarbital (Butisol)
mephobarbital (Mebaral)
pentobarbital (Nembutal)
phenobarbital

primidone (Mysoline)
secobarbital (Seconal)
talbutal (Lotusate)

Severity: ●●○
Probability: ●○○

USES: Griseofulvin is an antifungal agent used for ringworm infections of the skin, hair, and nails and also for certain types of bacterial infections. Barbiturates are used as sedatives or sleep inducers; phenobarbital and primidone are used for seizure disorders such as epilepsy.

EFFECT: The effect of griseofulvin may be decreased.

RESULT: The condition treated with griseofulvin may not be properly controlled.

WHAT TO DO: Use a higher dose of griseofulvin or take the two medications at separate times as warranted. Option: use alternative drugs.

123. ↓**guanethidine (Ismelin)**   **antidepressants, tricyclic**
                                        amitriptyline (Elavil, Endep)
                                        amoxapine (Asendin)
                                        clomipramine (Anafranil)
                                        desipramine
                                          Norpramin, Pertofrane
                                        doxepin (Adapin, Sinequan)
                                        imipramine (Tofranil)
                                        nortriptyline
                                          Aventyl, Pamelor
                                        protriptyline (Vivactil)
                                        trimipramine (Surmontil)

Severity: ●●○
Probability: ●●○

USES: Guanethidine is used for high blood pressure. Antidepressants are used for clinical depression.

EFFECT: The effect of guanethidine may be decreased.

RESULT: The blood pressure may not be properly controlled by guanethidine.

WHAT TO DO: Monitor blood pressure. Use an alternative to guanethidine as warranted.

124. ↓ **guanethidine (Ismelin)**   **appetite suppressants**
dextroamphetamine
  Biphetamine, Dexedrine
diethylpropion (Tenuate)
fenfluramine (Pondimin)
mazindol (Sanorex)
methamphetamine (Desoxyn)
phenmetrazine (Preludin)
phentermine (Ionamin)

Severity: ●●○
Probability: ●●○

USES: Guanethidine is used for high blood pressure. Appetite suppressants are used as short-term therapy for weight loss.

EFFECT: The effect of guanethidine may be reversed.

RESULT: The blood pressure may not be properly controlled by guanethidine.

WHAT TO DO: Monitor blood pressure. Use an alternative to guanethidine or stop the appetite suppressant as warranted.

125. ↓ **guanethidine (Ismelin)**   **phenothiazines**
acetophenazine (Tindal)
chlorpromazine (Thorazine)
fluphenazine (Permitil,
  Prolixin)
mesoridazine (Serentil)
perphenazine (Trilafon)
prochlorperazine
  Compazine
promazine (Sparine)
promethazine (Phenergan)
thioridazine (Mellaril)
trifluoperazine (Stelazine)

Severity: ●●○
Probability: ●●○

USES: Guanethidine is used for high blood pressure. Phenothiazines are antipsychotic drugs used for brain disorders such as schizophrenia, paranoia, and manic-depressive illness.

EFFECT: The effect of guanethidine may be reversed.

RESULT: The blood pressure may not be properly controlled by guanethidine.

WHAT TO DO: Monitor blood pressure. As options, use a higher dose of guanethidine or lower the dose of the phenothiazine, but do this cautiously. Use of an alternative to guanethidine may be warranted.

126. ↓ **guanethidine (Ismelin)**

sympathomimetics
↑Direct-acting
 dobutamine
 epinephrine
 methoxamine
 norepinephrine
 *phenylephrine
↓Mixed or indirect-acting
 dopamine
 *ephedrine
 mephentermine
 metaraminol
 *phenylpropanolamine
 *pseudoephedrine

Severity: ●●○
Probability: ●○○

USES: Guanethidine is used for high blood pressure. Sympathomimetics are used to treat shock; those marked by an asterisk are used in nonprescription cold and appetite suppressant products (read labels).

EFFECT: Both drug types are affected. The effect of guanethidine may be reversed. The effect of direct-acting sympathomimetics may be increased. The effect of mixed or indirect-acting sympathomimetics may be decreased.

RESULT: The blood pressure may not be properly controlled by guanethidine and heart beat irregularities may result.

WHAT TO DO: Closely monitor blood pressure. Stop the sympathomimetic or use an alternative to guanethidine as warranted.

127. ↓ **haloperidol (Haldol)**

anticholinergics
atropine
atropine/scopolamine/
  hyoscyamine
 Barbidonna, Donnatal
 Kinesed
belladonna

benztropine (Cogentin)
biperiden (Akineton)
clidinium (Quarzan)
dicyclomine (Bentyl)
glycopyrrolate (Robinul)
hyoscyamine (Anaspaz)
methantheline (Banthine)
orphenadrine (Pathilon)
oxybutynin (Ditropan)
procyclidine (Kemadrin)
propantheline (Pro-Banthine)
scopolamine (Transderm
   Scop)
tridihexethyl (Pathilon)
trihexyphenidyl (Artane)

Severity: ●●○
Probability: ●○○

USES: Haloperidol is an antipsychotic drug used for brain disorders such as schizophrenia, paranoia, and manic-depressive illness. Anticholinergics may be used for controlling the tremors resulting from Parkinson's disease or treatment with antipsychotic drugs; for stomach, digestive tract disorders; or for motion sickness.

EFFECT: Variable.

RESULT: Possible worsening of psychotic symptoms, development of tardive dyskinesia (involuntary movements), and decreased effect of haloperidol.

WHAT TO DO: Use anticholinergics only when expressly needed. Watch for symptoms and adjust the dose of haloperidol as needed. Stopping the anticholinergic may be necessary.

128. ↓ **haloperidol (Haldol)**   **carbamazepine
                                          (Epitol, Tegretol)**

Severity: ●●○
Probability: ●○○

USES: Haloperidol is an antipsychotic drug used for brain disorders such as schizophrenia, paranoia, and manic-depressive illness. Carbamazepine is used for seizure disorders such as epilepsy and for trigeminal neuralgia (severe pain in a facial nerve), also known as *tic douloureux*.

EFFECT: The effect of haloperidol may be decreased.

RESULT: The condition treated with haloperidol may not be properly controlled.

WHAT TO DO: Use a higher dose of haloperidol as needed.

129.   haloperidol (Haldol)   **lithium**
Cibalith-S, Eskalith, Lithane
Lithobid

Severity: ●●●
Probability: ●○○

USES: Haloperidol is an antipsychotic drug used for brain disorders such as schizophrenia, paranoia, and manic-depressive illness. Lithium is used for manic-depressive illness.

RESULT: Possible severe neurotoxic and extrapyramidal symptoms such as lethargy, fever, confusion, tremors.

WHAT TO DO: Closely monitor for symptoms. If an interaction is suspected, stop either drug.

130. ↑Insulin   **alcohol (ethanol)**
beer, liquor, wine

Severity: ●●●
Probability: ●●○

USES: Insulin is used for diabetes.

EFFECT: The effect of insulin may be increased.

RESULT: The blood sugar level may fall too low, resulting in hypoglycemia (low blood sugar) with symptoms such as nervousness, faintness, weakness, sweating, confusion, heart beat irregularities, rapid heart beats, loss of coordination, visual disturbances.

WHAT TO DO: Don't drink alcoholic beverages or drink moderately and with food if possible. Monitor closely for symptoms of hypoglycemia.

131. ↑Insulin   **beta blockers
                                                (nonselective)**
carteolol (Cartrol)
nadolol (Corgard)

penbutolol (Levatol)
pindolol (Visken)
propranolol (Inderal)
timolol (Blocadren)

Severity: ●●○
Probability: ●●●

USES: Insulin is used for diabetes. Beta blockers are used for high blood pressure, angina heart pain, and irregular heart beats; some have other uses such as for migraine headache and to calm the physical manifestations of "stage fright."

EFFECT: The effect of insulin may be increased.

RESULT: The blood sugar level may fall too low, resulting in hypoglycemia (low blood sugar) with symptoms such as nervousness, faintness, weakness, sweating, confusion, heart beat irregularities, rapid heart beats, loss of coordination, visual disturbances.

WHAT TO DO: Monitor closely for symptoms of hypoglycemia. Lower the insulin dose as needed. Be aware that the beta blocker can "hide" the warning symptoms of hypoglycemia. It may be best to substitute a noninteracting "cardioselective" beta blocker such as acebutolol (Sectral), atenolol (Tenormin), betaxolol (Kerlone), esmolol (Brevibloc), or metoprolol (Lopressor). A caution: at higher doses, these drugs also may interact.

132. ↑ Insulin   fenfluramine (Pondimin)

Severity: ●●○
Probability: ●●●

USES: Insulin is used for diabetes. Fenfluramine is an appetite suppressant used as short-term therapy for weight loss.

EFFECT: The effect of insulin may be increased.

RESULT: The blood sugar level may fall too low, resulting in hypoglycemia (low blood sugar) with symptoms such as nervousness, faintness, weakness, sweating, confusion, heart beat irregularities, rapid heart beats, loss of coordination, visual disturbances.

WHAT TO DO: Monitor blood glucose levels and watch for symptoms of hypoglycemia. Lower the insulin dose as needed.

133. ↑ Insulin

MAO Inhibitors
isocarboxazid (Marplan)
pargyline (Eutonyl)
phenelzine (Nardil)
tranylcypromine (Parnate)

Severity: ●●○
Probability: ●●●

USES: Insulin is used for diabetes. MAO inhibitors are used for some cases of clinical depression.

EFFECT: The effect of insulin may be increased.

RESULT: The blood sugar level may fall too low, resulting in hypoglycemia (low blood sugar) with symptoms such as nervousness, faintness, weakness, sweating, confusion, heart beat irregularities, rapid heart beats, loss of coordination, visual disturbances.

WHAT TO DO: Monitor blood glucose levels and watch for symptoms of hypoglycemia. Lower the insulin dose as needed.

134. ↑ Insulin

salicylates
aspirin
  Alka Seltzer, Anacin,
  Ascriptin, Aspergum, Bayer
  Bufferin, Cama, Ecotrin
  Empirin, Measurin,
  Momentum, Persistin,
  St. Joseph
bismuth subsalicylate
  Pepto Bismol
choline salicylate (Arthropan)
magnesium salicylate
  Doan's
salsalate (Disalcid)
sodium salicylate (Uracel)
sodium thiosalicylate (Tusal)

Severity: ●●○
Probability: ●●○

USES: Insulin is used for diabetes. Salicylates such as aspirin are used for arthritic-type conditions and for general pain, fever, and inflammation.

EFFECT: The effect of insulin may be increased.

RESULT: The blood sugar level may fall too low, resulting in hypoglycemia (low blood sugar) with symptoms such as nervousness, faintness, weakness, sweating, confusion, heart beat irregularities, rapid heart beats, loss of coordination, visual disturbances.

WHAT TO DO: Monitor blood glucose levels and watch for symptoms of hypoglycemia. Lower the insulin dose as needed.

135. ↓**Iron**

ferrous fumarate
ferrous gluconate
ferrous sulfate
iron polysaccharide
Brand names:
Caltrate, Chromagen, Feosol
Feostat, Ferancee, Fergon
Fero-Folic-500, Fero-Grad-50
Ferralet, Ferro-Sequel
Fosfree, Hemocyte, Hytinic
Iberet, Ircon, Iromin-G
Mission Prenatal, Mol-Iron
Natalins Rx, Poly-Vi-Flor
Pramet FA, Pramilet FA
Simron, Slow Fe, Stuartinic
Trinsicon, Zenate

antacids

AlternaGEL, Amphojel
Camalox, Chooz, Delcid
Di-Gel, Gaviscon
Gelusil, Kudrox
Maalox, Mylanta, Riopan
Rolaids, Titralac, Tums

Severity: ●●○
Probability: ●○○

USES: Iron is an essential mineral available in numerous over-the-counter vitamin/mineral products (read product labels for the ingredients listed above). Antacids are used for stomach problems associated with too much stomach acid.

EFFECT: The effect of iron may be decreased.

RESULT: The full benefit of the iron supplement may not be realized.

WHAT TO DO: Take the two medications at separate times, as far apart as feasible.

136. ↓**Iron**

ferrous fumarate
ferrous gluconate
ferrous sulfate
iron polysaccharide

chloramphenicol

Chloromycetin

Brand names:
Caltrate, Chromagen, Feosol
Feostat, Ferancee, Fergon
Fero-Folic-500, Fero-Grad-50
Ferralet, Ferro-Sequel
Fosfree, Hemocyte, Hytinic
Iberet, Ircon, Iromin-G
Mission Prenatal, Mol-Iron
Natalins Rx, Poly-Vi-Flor
Pramet FA, Pramilet FA
Simron, Slow Fe, Stuartinic
Trinsicon, Zenate

Severity: ●●○
Probability: ●○○

USES: Iron is an essential mineral available in numerous over-the-counter vitamin/mineral products (read product labels for the ingredients listed above). Chloramphenicol is an antibiotic used for microbial infections.

EFFECT: The response to iron therapy may be decreased.

RESULT: Increased risk of developing anemia.

WHAT TO DO: It's probably best not to take chloramphenicol if you are taking an iron supplement for iron-deficiency anemia. If possible, take an alternative antibiotic.

137.	**Isoniazid**	**rifampin**
	INH	Rifadin
	Laniazid	Rifamate
	Nydrazid	Rimactane
	Rimactane	Rimactane/INH
	Rimactane/INH	

Severity: ●●●
Probability: ●○○

USES: Isoniazid is used for tuberculosis. Rifampin is a specialized antibiotic used for tuberculosis and may also be given to suspected meningitis carriers.

RESULT: Higher risk of liver toxicity than with either drug alone.

WHAT TO DO: Close monitoring and liver function tests are warranted. If problems arise, stop one or both drugs.

138. ↓ **ketoconazole (Nizoral)**   ↓ **rifampin**
Rifadin
Rifamate
Rimactane
Rimactane/INH

     Severity: ●●○
Probability: ●○○

USES: Ketoconazole is used for systemic fungal infections such as thrush and for fungal infections of the skin and nails. Rifampin is a specialized antibiotic used for tuberculosis and may also be given to suspected meningitis carriers.

EFFECT: The effect of both drugs may be decreased.

RESULT: The conditions treated may not be properly controlled.

WHAT TO DO: Monitor blood levels of both drugs and the patient's antibiotic response. Avoid this combination if possible.

139.   **levodopa**   **MAO inhibitors**
          (Larodopa, Sinemet)

                                  isocarboxazid (Marplan)
                                  pargyline (Eutonyl)
                                  phenelzine (Nardil)
                                  tranylcypromine (Parnate)

     Severity: ●●●
Probability: ●●●

USES: Levodopa is used for Parkinson's disease. MAO inhibitors are used for some cases of clinical depression.

RESULT: This combination may cause an abrupt rise in blood pressure with symptoms such as headache, fever, visual disturbances, and confusion.

WHAT TO DO: Avoid this dangerous combination.

140. ↓ **levodopa**   **phenytoin (Dilantin)**
          (Larodopa, Sinemet)

                                  ethotoin (Peganone)
                                  mephenytoin (Mesantoin)

     Severity: ●●○
Probability: ●○○

USES: Levodopa is used for Parkinson's disease. Phenytoin is an anticonvulsant used for seizure disorders such as epilepsy.

EFFECT: The effect of levodopa may be decreased.

RESULT: The condition treated with levodopa may not be properly controlled.

WHAT TO DO: Use a higher dose of levodopa as needed. It may be best to avoid using phenytoin.

141. ↓ levodopa (Larodopa,   vitamin B-6 (pyridoxine)
        Sinemet)

      Severity: ●●○
Probability: ●●●

USES: Levodopa is used for Parkinson's disease. Vitamin B-6 is an essential vitamin.

EFFECT: The effect of levodopa may be decreased.

RESULT: The condition treated with levodopa may not be properly controlled.

WHAT TO DO: Avoid taking vitamin B-6 with straight levodopa. Instead, use a levodopa/carbidopa preparation such as Sinemet, which is negligibly affected by vitamin B-6.

142. ↑ lithium   carbamazepine
                         (Epitol, Tegretol)

     Cibalith-S
     Eskalith
     Lithane
     Lithobid

      Severity: ●●○
Probability: ●○○

USES: Lithium is used for manic-depressive illness. Carbamazepine is used for seizure disorders such as epilepsy and for trigeminal neuralgia (severe pain in a facial nerve), also known as *tic douloureux*.

EFFECT: The effect of lithium may be increased.

RESULT: Increased risk of toxicity even though lithium blood levels may not be significantly increased. Symptoms of toxicity include dizziness, nausea, confusion, weakness, lethargy, dry mouth, loss of appetite, stomach or abdominal pain, loss of coordination.

WHAT TO DO: Monitor for symptoms and stop either drug as needed.

143. ↑**lithium**   **diuretics, loop**
     Cibalith-S   bumetanide (Bumex)
     Eskalith   ethacrynic acid (Edecrin)
     Lithane   furosemide (Lasix)
     Lithobid

   Severity: ●●○
Probability: ●○○

USES: Lithium is used for manic-depressive illness. Diuretics are used to rid the body of excess fluid—this makes them effective in treating congestive heart failure, high blood pressure, cirrhosis of the liver, and kidney dysfunction.

EFFECT: The effect of lithium may be increased.

RESULT: Increased risk of toxicity with symptoms such as dizziness, nausea, confusion, weakness, lethargy, dry mouth, loss of appetite, stomach or abdominal pain, loss of coordination.

WHAT TO DO: Monitor lithium blood levels and symptoms, and adjust the lithium dose as needed.

144. ↑**lithium**   **diuretics, thiazide**
     Cibalith-S   bendroflumethiazide
     Eskalith   Naturetin
     Lithane   benzthiazide (Aquatag)
     Lithobid   chlorothiazide (Diuril)
                                        chlorthalidone (Hygroton)
                                        cyclothiazide (Anhydron)
                                        hydrochlorothiazide
                                           Esidrix, HydroDiuril
                                        hydroflumethiazide (Saluron)
                                        indapamide (Lozol)
                                        methyclothiazide (Enduron)
                                        metolazone (Diulo,
                                           Zaroxolyn)
                                        polythiazide (Renese)
                                        quinethazone (Hydromox)
                                        trichlormethiazide (Naqua)

   Severity: ●●○
Probability: ●●●

USES: Lithium is used for manic-depressive illness. Diuretics are used to rid the body of excess fluid—this makes them effective in treating congestive heart failure, high blood pressure, cirrhosis of the liver, and kidney dysfunction.

EFFECT: The effect of lithium may be increased.

RESULT: Increased risk of lithium toxicity with symptoms such as dizziness, nausea, confusion, weakness, lethargy, dry mouth, loss of appetite, stomach or abdominal pain, loss of coordination.

WHAT TO DO: Monitor lithium blood levels and symptoms, and adjust the lithium dose as needed.

145. **lithium**   **iodide salts**
Cibalith-S   calcium iodide
Eskalith   hydrogen iodide
Lithane   Hydriodic Acid
Lithobid   iodide
                                       iodinated glycerol
                                          Organidin
                                       iodine
                                       potassium iodide (SSKI)
                                       sodium iodide

Severity: ●●○
Probability: ●○○

USES: Lithium is used for manic-depressive illness. Iodide salts are used as expectorants (agents which help liquefy mucus) in chronic lung diseases, for thyroid blocking in a radiation emergency, or with an antithyroid drug in hyperthyroid patients in preparation for thyroidectomy or for thyrotoxic crisis.

RESULT: Increased risk of hypothyroidism (deficiency of thyroid) and goiter (enlargement of the thyroid gland).

WHAT TO DO: Avoid this combination if possible.

146. ↑**lithium**   **methyldopa**
                                          (Aldomet, Aldoril)
Cibalith-S
Eskalith
Lithane
Lithobid

Severity: ●●○
Probability: ●○○

USES: Lithium is used for manic-depressive illness. Methyldopa is used for high blood pressure.

EFFECT: The effect of lithium may be increased.

RESULT: Increased risk of toxicity even though lithium blood levels may not be significantly increased. Symptoms of toxicity include dizziness, nausea, confusion, weakness, lethargy, dry mouth, loss of appetite, stomach or abdominal pain, loss of coordination.

WHAT TO DO: Monitor for symptoms and stop either drug as needed.

147. ↑ **lithium**
   Cibalith-S
   Eskalith
   Lithane
   Lithobid

NSAIDs
diclofenac (Voltaren)
ibuprofen (Motrin, Rufen)
   Advil, Haltran, Medipren,
   Midol 200, Pamprin-IB,
   Nuprin, Trendar
indomethacin (Indocin)
naproxen (Anaprox,
   Naprosyn)
piroxicam (Feldenc)

Severity: ●●○
Probability: ●○○

USES: Lithium is used for manic-depressive illness. NSAIDs (nonsteroidal antiinflammatory drugs) are used for pain and inflammation in arthritic-type conditions and for general pain and inflammation.

EFFECT: The effect of lithium may be increased.

RESULT: Increased risk of lithium toxicity with symptoms such as dizziness, nausea, confusion, weakness, lethargy, dry mouth, loss of appetite, stomach or abdominal pain, loss of coordination. (It has not been determined whether NSAIDs other than those listed above interact.)

WHAT TO DO: Monitor lithium blood levels and symptoms, and adjust the lithium dose as needed.

148. ↓ **lithium**
   Cibalith-S
   Eskalith
   Lithane
   Lithobid

theophyllines
aminophylline
   Somophyllin
dyphylline
   Dilor, Lufyllin

oxtriphylline
  Choledyl
theophylline
  Aerolate, Bronkodyl,
  Bronkaid, Constant-T,
  Elixophyllin, Marax,
  Mudrane, Primatene,
  Quibron, Respbid, Slo-bid,
  Slo-Phyllin, T-PHYL,
  Tedral, Theo-24, Theo-Dur,
  Theo-Organidin, Theobid,
  Theolair, Theospan-SR,
  Theostat 80, Uniphyl

Severity: ●●○
Probability: ●○○

USES: Lithium is used for manic-depressive illness. Theophylline is used for asthma and for bronchospasm associated with chronic bronchitis and emphysema.

EFFECT: The effect of lithium may be decreased.

RESULT: The condition treated with lithium may not be properly controlled.

WHAT TO DO: Monitor lithium blood levels and clinical response, and adjust the lithium dose as needed.

149. ↓ **lithium**   **urinary alkalinizers**
  Cibalith-S   potassium citrate
  Eskalith   Alka-Seltzer
  Lithane   K-Lyte
  Lithobid   sodium acetate
                                        sodium bicarbonate
                                          Alka-Seltzer
                                          Citrocarbonate
                                        sodium citrate
                                          Alka-Seltzer
                                        sodium lactate
                                        tromethamine

Severity: ●●○
Probability: ●○○

USES: Lithium is used for manic-depressive illness. Urinary alkalinizers are used in some antacids and in some potassium supplement products.

EFFECT: The effect of lithium may be decreased.

RESULT: The condition treated with lithium may not be properly controlled.

WHAT TO DO: Avoid regular use of urinary alkalinizers.

---

150.   meperidine (Demerol)

MAO Inhibitors
isocarboxazid (Marplan)
pargyline (Eutonyl)
phenelzine (Nardil)
tranylcypromine (Parnate)

Severity: ●●●
Probability: ●○○

USES: Meperidine is a narcotic used for moderate to severe pain. MAO inhibitors are used for some cases of clinical depression.

RESULT: Increased risk of severe adverse effects such as excitation, seizures, fever, sweating, breathing difficulties, low blood pressure, loss of consciousness, coma. The risk of adverse effects may persist for several weeks after stopping the MAO inhibitor.

WHAT TO DO: Avoid this dangerous combination.

---

151.   meperidine (Demerol)

phenothiazines
acetophenazine (Tindal)
chlorpromazine (Thorazine)
fluphenazine (Permitil,
   Prolixin)
mesoridazine (Serentil)
perphenazine (Trilafon)
prochlorperazine
   Compazine
promazine (Sparine)
promethazine (Phenergan)
thioridazine (Mellaril)
trifluoperazine (Stelazine)

Severity: ●●○
Probability: ●●○

USES: Meperidine is a narcotic used for moderate to severe pain. Phenothiazines are antipsychotic drugs used for brain disorders such as schizophrenia, paranoia, and manic-depressive illness.

RESULT: Increased risk of excessive sedation and low blood pressure. Narcotic pain relievers other than meperidine may also interact.

WHAT TO DO: Avoid this combination if possible.

152. ↓**methadone (Dolophine)**   **phenytoin (Dilantin)**
ethotoin (Peganone)
mephenytoin (Mesantoin)

Severity: ●○○
Probability: ●○○

USES: Methadone is a narcotic pain reliever also used for detoxification treatment of narcotic addiction. Phenytoin is an anticonvulsant used for seizure disorders such as epilepsy.

EFFECT: The effect of methadone may be decreased.

RESULT: The condition treated with methadone may not be properly controlled.

WHAT TO DO: Use a higher dose of methadone as warranted.

153. ↓**methadone (Dolophine)**   **rifampin**
Rifadin
Rifamate
Rimactane
Rimactane/INH

Severity: ●○○
Probability: ●○○

USES: Methadone is a narcotic pain reliever also used for detoxification treatment of narcotic addiction. Rifampin is a specialized antibiotic used for tuberculosis and may also be given to suspected meningitis carriers.

EFFECT: The effect of methadone may be decreased.

RESULT: The condition treated with methadone may not be properly controlled.

WHAT TO DO: Use a higher dose of methadone as warranted.

154. ↓ **methadone (Dolophine)**

urinary acidifiers
ammonium chloride
  Ipsatol Expectorant Syrup
  P-V-Tussin Syrup
  Quelidrine Syrup
potassium acid phosphate
  K-Phos
  K-Phos No. 2
  Thiacide
sodium acid phosphate
  K-Phos No. 2
  Uroqid-Acid
  Uroqid-Acid No. 2

Severity: ●○○
Probability: ●○○

USES: Methadone is a narcotic pain reliever also used for detoxification treatment of narcotic addiction. Urinary acidifiers: ammonium chloride is an expectorant (agent which liquefies mucus) and is used in some cough syrups; potassium acid phosphate and sodium acid phosphate are used to make the urine more acidic.

EFFECT: The effect of methadone may be decreased.

WHAT TO DO: This is a "good" interaction when it is used to treat methadone overdose.

155. ↑ **methotrexate**
     (Folex, Mexate)

probenecid

Benemid
ColBenemid

Severity: ●●●
Probability: ●●○

USES: Methotrexate is used as cancer chemotherapy, for severe psoriasis, and has shown value in treatment of rheumatoid arthritis, psoriatic arthritis, and Reiter's syndrome (an inflammatory disease occurring mainly in young men). Probenecid is used for gout and gouty arthritis.

EFFECT: The effect of methotrexate may be increased.

RESULT: Increased risk of methotrexate toxicity.

WHAT TO DO: Monitor methotrexate blood levels and do other laboratory tests as warranted. Use a lower dose when necessary.

156. ↑methotrexate   **salicylates**
(Folex, Mexate)

aspirin
  Alka Seltzer, Anacin
  Ascriptin, Aspergum, Bayer
  Bufferin, Cama, Ecotrin
  Empirin, Measurin
  Momentum, Persistin
  St. Joseph
bismuth subsalicylate
  Pepto Bismol
choline salicylate (Arthropan)
magnesium salicylate (Doan's)
salsalate (Disalcid)
sodium salicylate (Uracel)
sodium thiosalicylate (Tusal)

Severity: ●●●
Probability: ●○○

USES: Methotrexate is used as cancer chemotherapy, for severe psoriasis, and has shown value in treatment of rheumatoid arthritis, psoriatic arthritis, and Reiter's syndrome (an inflammatory disease occurring mainly in young men). Salicylates such as aspirin are used for arthritic-type conditions and for general pain, fever, and inflammation.

EFFECT: The effect of methotrexate may be increased.

RESULT: Increased risk of methotrexate toxicity.

WHAT TO DO: Monitor methotrexate blood levels and do other laboratory tests as warranted. Use a lower dose when necessary.

157. methyldopa   **beta blockers**
(Aldomet, Aldoril)   **(nonselective)**
carteolol (Cartrol)
nadolol (Corgard)
penbutolol (Levatol)
pindolol (Visken)
propranolol (Inderal)
timolol (Blocadren)

Severity: ●●●
Probability: ●○○

USES: Methyldopa is used for high blood pressure. Beta blockers are used for high blood pressure, angina heart pain, and irregular heart beats. Some have other uses, such as in the prevention of migraine headache and to calm the physical manifestations of "stage fright."

RESULT: Increased risk of a high blood pressure crisis with adverse symptoms such as restlessness and irritability, tremors, rapid heart beat, headache, nausea, fever, visual disturbances. (Note: This interaction appears more likely to occur in patients who are also taking an indirect-acting sympathomimetic (e.g., phenylpropanolamine, pseudoephedrine—used in many nonprescription cold and cough products and in appetite suppressants (read product labels).

WHAT TO DO: Monitor blood pressure and symptoms, and treat an adverse episode with phentolamine (Regitine).

158. ↓ **metronidazole**
Flagyl
Mctryl
Protostat

barbiturates
amobarbital (Amytal)
aprobarbital (Alurate)
butabarbital (Butisol)
butalbital
mephobarbital (Mebaral)
pentobarbital (Nembutal)
phenobarbital
primidone (Mysoline)
secobarbital (Seconal)
talbutal (Lotusate)

Severity: ●●○
Probability: ●○○

USES: Metronidazole is used for trichomoniasis, a type of vaginitis, and for acute amoebic dysentery. Barbiturates are used as sedatives or sleep inducers; phenobarbital and primidone are used for seizure disorders such as epilepsy.

EFFECT: The effect of metronidazole may be decreased.

RESULT: The condition treated with metronidazole may not be properly controlled.

WHAT TO DO: Monitor clinical response and use a higher dose of metronidazole when needed.

159. ↓ **mexiletine (Mexitil)**   **phenytoin (Dilantin)**
                                              ethotoin (Peganone)
                                              mephenytoin (Mesantoin)

Severity: ●●○
Probability: ●○○

USES: Mexiletine is used for heart beat irregularities of the ventricular type. Phenytoin is an anticonvulsant used for seizure disorders such as epilepsy.

EFFECT: The effect of mexiletine may be decreased.

RESULT: The condition treated with mexiletine may not be properly controlled.

WHAT TO DO: Monitor mexiletine blood levels and clinical response, and use a higher dose of mexiletine as needed.

160. ↑ **nifedipine**   **cimetidine (Tagamet)**
          (Adalat, Procardia)

Severity: ●●○
Probability: ●○○

USES: Nifedipine is a calcium channel blocker used for high blood pressure, angina heart pain, and irregular heart beats. Cimetidine and ranitidine are used for duodenal and gastric ulcers.

EFFECT: The effect of nifedipine may be increased.

RESULT: Increased risk of adverse effects such as low blood pressure, rapid heart beat.

WHAT TO DO: Watch for symptoms and lower the dose of nifedipine as needed.

161. ↓ **nitrofurantoin**   **magnesium**
          (Macrodantin)
                                              antacids (various)
                                              milk of magnesia

Severity: ●○○
Probability: ●○○

USES: Nitrofurantoin is used for urinary tract infections. Magnesium salts are found in numerous over-the-counter antacid products (read product labels) and in milk of magnesia, a laxative.

EFFECT: The effect of nitrofurantoin may be decreased.

RESULT: The condition treated with nitrofurantoin may not be properly controlled.

WHAT TO DO: Avoid this combination if possible. Taking the two medications as far apart as feasible or switching to an aluminum-only antacid are options. Aluminum-only antacids include AlternaGEL, Aludrox, and Amphojel.

162. ↓**penicillamine, oral**   **food**
    Cuprimine
    Depen

    Severity: ●●○
Probability: ●○○

USES: Penicillamine is used for Wilson's disease (a genetic disorder causing an abnormality in copper metabolism), cystinuria (amino acids in the urine), and severe rheumatoid arthritis.

EFFECT: The effect of penicillamine may be decreased.

RESULT: The condition treated with penicillamine may not be properly controlled.

WHAT TO DO: Take penicillamine on an empty stomach at least an hour before or two hours after food or milk.

163. ↓**penicillamine, oral**   **aluminum**
    Cuprimine   aluminum carbonate
    Depen   aluminum hydroxide
                                       aluminum phosphate
                                       attapulgite
                                       dihydroxyaluminum
                                          aminoacetate
                                       dihydroxyaluminum sodium
                                         carbonate
                                       kaolin
                                       magaldrate
                                       Brand names:
                                          AlternaGEL, Aludrox
                                          Amphojel, Basaljel,
                                          Camalox, Creamalin, Delcid
                                          Diasorb, Di-Gel, Gaviscon
                                          Gelusil, Kaopectate

Kolantyl, Kudrox, Maalox
Mylanta, Phosphaljel
Rheaban, Riopan, Rolaids
Tempo, WinGel
sucralfate (Carafate)

Severity: ●●○
Probability: ●●○

USES: Penicillamine is used for Wilson's disease (a genetic disorder causing an abnormality in copper metabolism), cystinuria (amino acids in the urine), and severe rheumatoid arthritis. Aluminum salts are used in various over-the-counter antacids (read product labels); in Kaopectate (for diarrhea); and in sucralfate (Carafate), a prescription product used for stomach ulcers.

EFFECT: The effect of penicillamine may be decreased.

RESULT: The condition treated with penicillamine may not be properly controlled.

WHAT TO DO: Take these two types of medications as far apart as feasible. Use a higher dose of penicillamine as warranted.

164.   ↓penicillamine, oral   **Iron**
Cuprimine   ferrous fumarate
Depen   ferrous gluconate
                                       ferrous sulfate
                                       iron polysaccharide
                                       Brand names:
                                         Caltrate, Chromagen, Feosol
                                         Feostat, Ferancee, Fergon
                                         Fero-Folic-500, Fero-Grad-50
                                         Ferralet, Ferro-Sequel
                                         Fosfree, Hemocyte, Hytinic
                                         Iberet, Ircon, Iromin-G
                                         Mission Prenatal, Mol-Iron
                                         Natalins Rx, Poly-Vi-Flor
                                         Pramet FA, Pramilet FA
                                         Simron, Slow Fe, Stuartinic
                                         Trinsicon, Zenate

Severity: ●●○
Probability: ●●○

USES: Penicillamine is used for Wilson's disease (a genetic disorder causing an abnormality in copper metabolism), cystinuria (amino acids in the urine), and severe rheumatoid arthritis. Iron is an essential mineral available in numerous over-the-counter vitamin/mineral products (read product labels for the ingredients listed above).

EFFECT: The effect of penicillamine may be decreased.

RESULT: The condition treated with penicillamine may not be properly controlled.

WHAT TO DO: Take these two preparations as far apart as feasible.

---

165. ↓**penicillamine, oral**   **magnesium**
       Cuprimine   antacids (various)
       Depen   milk of magnesia

      Severity: ●○○
Probability: ●○○

USES: Penicillamine is used for Wilson's disease (a genetic disorder causing an abnormality in copper metabolism), cystinuria (amino acids in the urine), and severe rheumatoid arthritis. Magnesium salts are found in numerous over-the-counter antacid products (read product labels) and in milk of magnesia, a laxative.

EFFECT: The effect of penicillamine may be decreased.

RESULT: The condition treated with penicillamine may not be properly controlled.

WHAT TO DO: Take these two preparations as far apart as feasible.

---

166.   **penicillins**   **allopurinol (Zyloprim)**
       ampicillin
         Amcill, Omnipen,
         Polycillin, Principen

      Severity: ●●○
Probability: ●○○

USES: Ampicillin is an antibiotic used for microbial infections. Allopurinol is used for gout and in certain types of cancer therapy.

RESULT: Increased risk of ampicillin-caused skin rash.

WHAT TO DO: Monitor for allergic-like skin rashes and lower the dose of allopurinol (or discontinue this combination) as warranted.

167. ↓penicillins   tetracyclines
      amdinocillin (Coactin)   demeclocycline (Declomycin)
      amoxicillin (Amoxil, Polymox)   doxycycline
      ampicillin   Doryx, Vibramycin
        Amcill, Omnipen,   Vibra-tab
        Polycillin, Principen   methacycline (Rondomycin)
      azlocillin (Azlin)   minocycline (Minocin)
      bacampicillin (Spectrobid)   oxytetracycline (Terramycin)
      carbenicillin   tetracycline
        Geopen, Geocillin   Achromycin V, Sumycin
      cloxacillin (Tegopen)
      dicloxacillin (Dynapen)
      methicillin (Staphcillin)
      mezlocillin (Mezlin)
      nafcillin (Unipen)
      oxacillin (Prostaphlin)
      penicillin G (Pentids)
      penicillin V
        Betapen-VK, Pen Vee K,
        Veetids
      piperacillin (Pipracil)
      ticarcillin (Ticar)

   Severity: ●●●
   Probability: ●○○

USES: Penicillin and tetracycline are antibiotics used for microbial
infections.

EFFECT: The effect of penicillin may be decreased.

RESULT: The infection treated with penicillin may not be properly
controlled.

WHAT TO DO: Avoid this combination if possible.

168. ↓penicillins, oral   food
      ampicillin
        Amcill, Omnipen,
        Polycillin, Principen
      bacampicillin (Spectrobid)
      carbenicillin
        Geopen, Geocillin
      cloxacillin (Tegopen)
      dicloxacillin (Dynapen)

nafcillin (Unipen)
oxacillin (Prostaphlin)
penicillin G (Pentids)

Severity: ●●○
Probability: ●○○

USES: Penicillin is an antibiotic used for microbial infections.

EFFECT: The effect of penicillin may be decreased.

RESULT: The infection treated with penicillin may not be properly controlled.

WHAT TO DO: Take the penicillins in the above list at least one hour before or two hours after meals.

169. ↑**pentoxifylline (Trental)**   **cimetidine (Tagamet)**

Severity: ●○○
Probability: ●○○

USES: Pentoxifylline is used for intermittent claudication (severe pain in calf muscles during activity, a condition resulting from inadequate blood supply to the area). Cimetidine is used for duodenal and gastric ulcers.

EFFECT: The effect of pentoxifylline may be increased.

RESULT: Increased risk of adverse effects such as dyspnea (difficult breathing), edema (excess body fluid), low blood pressure, loss of appetite, dry mouth, thirst, constipation, anxiety, confusion.

WHAT TO DO: Lower the dose of pentoxifylline as needed. Option: use a noninteracting alternative to cimetidine such as famotidine (Pepcid) or nizatidine (Axid).

170. ↓**phenothiazines**   **anticholinergics**

acetophenazine (Tindal)   atropine
chlorpromazine (Thorazine)   atropine/scopolamine/
fluphenazine (Permitil,   hyoscyamine
   Prolixin)   Barbidonna, Donnatal
mesoridazine (Serentil)   Kinesed
perphenazine (Trilafon)   belladonna
prochlorperazine   benztropine (Cogentin)
   Compazine   biperiden (Akineton)

promazine (Sparine)
promethazine (Phenergan)
thioridazine (Mellaril)
trifluoperazine (Stelazine)

clidinium (Quarzan)
dicyclomine (Bentyl)
glycopyrrolate (Robinul)
hyoscyamine (Anaspaz)
methantheline (Banthine)
orphenadrine (Disipal)
oxybutynin (Ditropan)
procyclidine (Kemadrin)
propantheline (Pro-Banthine)
scopolamine (Transderm
    Scop)
tridihexethyl (Pathilon)
trihexyphenidyl (Artane)

Severity: ●●○
Probability: ●○○

USES: Phenothiazines are antipsychotic drugs used for brain disorders such as schizophrenia, paranoia, and manic-depressive illness. Anticholinergics may be used for controlling the tremors resulting from Parkinson's disease or treatment with antipsychotic drugs; for stomach, digestive tract disorders; or for motion sickness.

EFFECT: Variable.

RESULT: Possible worsening of psychotic symptoms, development of tardive dyskinesia (involuntary movements), and decreased effect of the phenothiazine.

WHAT TO DO: Use anticholinergics only when expressly needed. Watch for symptoms and adjust the phenothiazine dose as needed. Stop the anticholinergic if necessary.

171. ↓**phenothiazines**
acetophenazine (Tindal)
chlorpromazine (Thorazine)
fluphenazine (Permitil,
    Prolixin)
mesoridazine (Serentil)
perphenazine (Trilafon)
prochlorperazine
    Compazine
promazine (Sparine)
promethazine (Phenergan)
thioridazine (Mellaril)
trifluoperazine (Stelazine)

lithium
Cibalith-S
Eskalith
Lithane
Lithobid

Severity: ●●○
Probability: ●○○

USES: Phenothiazines are antipsychotic drugs used for brain disorders such as schizophrenia, paranoia, and manic-depressive illness. Lithium is used for manic-depressive illness.

EFFECT: The effect of the phenothiazine may be decreased. In rarer cases, severe neurotoxicity has occurred in acute manic patients, especially with the phenothiazine thioridazine.

RESULT: The condition treated may not be properly controlled. Symptoms of severe neurotoxicity include disorientation, delirium, seizures.

WHAT TO DO: Monitor for adverse symptoms and lower the dose of one or both drugs or discontinue this combination.

172. ↓ **phenylbutazone** **barbiturates**
     (Butazolidin)
     oxyphenbutazone   amobarbital (Amytal)
                                      aprobarbital (Alurate)
                                      butabarbital (Butisol)
                                      butalbital
                                      mephobarbital (Mebaral)
                                      pentobarbital (Nembutal)
                                      phenobarbital
                                      primidone (Mysoline)
                                      secobarbital (Seconal)
                                      talbutal (Lotusate)

Severity: ●○○
Probability: ●○○

USES: Phenylbutazone is used for the pain and inflammation of arthritic-type conditions. Barbiturates are used as sedatives or sleep inducers; phenobarbital and primidone are used for seizure disorders such as epilepsy.

EFFECT: The effect of phenylbutazone may be decreased.

RESULT: The condition treated with phenylbutazone may not be properly controlled.

WHAT TO DO: Use an alternative to one of the two interacting drugs as warranted.

173. ↑ **phenytoin (Dilantin)**   **amiodarone
                                                          (Cordarone)**

ethotoin (Peganone)
mephenytoin (Mesantoin)

Severity: ●●○
Probability: ●○○

USES: Phenytoin is an anticonvulsant drug used for seizure disorders
such as epilepsy. Amiodarone is used for heart beat irregularities of
the ventricular type.

EFFECT: The effect of phenytoin may be increased.

RESULT: Increased risk of phenytoin toxicity with symptoms such
as nystagmus (uncontrolled movement of the eyeballs), double vision, loss of coordination, slurred speech, tremor, lethargy, nausea,
vomiting.

WHAT TO DO: Monitor phenytoin blood levels and symptoms, and
lower the phenytoin dose as needed.

174. ↓ **phenytoin (Dilantin)**   **antineoplastic agents**
ethotoin (Peganone)   bleomycin (Blenoxane)
mephenytoin (Mesantoin)   carmustine (BiCNU)
                                                         cisplatin (Platinol)
                                                         methotrexate (Folex, Mexate)
                                                         vinblastine (Velban)

Severity: ●●○
Probability: ●○○

USES: Phenytoin is an anticonvulsant drug used for seizure disorders
such as epilepsy. Antineoplastic agents are used in cancer chemotherapy.

EFFECT: The effect of phenytoin may be decreased.

RESULT: The condition treated with phenytoin may not be properly
controlled.

WHAT TO DO: Monitor clinical response and use a higher dose of
phenytoin as needed.

175. ↑ **phenytoin (Dilantin)**   ↓ **carbamazepine
                                                (Epitol, Tegretol)**

ethotoin (Peganone)
mephenytoin (Mesantoin)

Severity: ●●○
Probability: ●○○

USES: Phenytoin and carbamazepine are both anticonvulsant drugs used for seizure disorders such as epilepsy. Carbamazepine is also used for certain types of neuralgia (nerve pain).

EFFECT: The effect of phenytoin may be variable. The effect of carbamazepine may be decreased.

RESULT: The conditions treated with the drugs may not be properly controlled.

WHAT TO DO: Monitor the blood levels of both drugs and observe clinical response. Adjust dosages as warranted.

176. ↑ **phenytoin (Dilantin)**   ↓ **chloramphenicol**
       ethotoin (Peganone)   Chloromycetin
       mephenytoin (Mesantoin)

Severity: ●●○
Probability: ●○○

USES: Phenytoin is an anticonvulsant drug used for seizure disorders such as epilepsy. Chloramphenicol is an antibiotic used for microbial infections.

EFFECT: The effect of phenytoin may be increased. Also, the effect of chloramphenicol may be decreased.

RESULT: Increased risk of phenytoin toxicity with symptoms such as nystagmus (uncontrolled movement of the eyeballs), double vision, loss of coordination, slurred speech, tremor, lethargy, nausea, vomiting. Also, the infection treated with chloramphenicol may not be properly controlled.

WHAT TO DO: Monitor blood levels of both drugs and watch for symptoms of phenytoin toxicity. Adjust doses as needed.

177. ↑ **phenytoin (Dilantin)**   **cimetidine (Tagamet)**
       ethotoin (Peganone)
       mephenytoin (Mesantoin)

Severity: ●●○
Probability: ●●●

USES: Phenytoin is an anticonvulsant drug used for seizure disorders such as epilepsy. Cimetidine is used for duodenal and gastric ulcers.

EFFECT: The effect of phenytoin may be increased.

RESULT: Increased risk of phenytoin toxicity with symptoms such as nystagmus (uncontrolled movement of the eyeballs), double vision, loss of coordination, slurred speech, tremor, lethargy, nausea, vomiting.

WHAT TO DO: Monitor phenytoin blood levels and symptoms, and lower the dose of phenytoin as needed.

178. ↓ **phenytoin (Dilantin)**   **diazoxide (Proglycem)**
        ethotoin (Peganone)
        mephenytoin (Mesantoin)

        Severity: ●●○
Probability: ●○○

USES: Phenytoin is an anticonvulsant drug used for seizure disorders such as epilepsy. Diazoxide is used to manage hypoglycemia (low blood sugar) associated with a variety of conditions which cause hyperinsulinism (production of too much insulin by the body).

EFFECT: The effect of phenytoin may be decreased.

RESULT: The condition treated with phenytoin may not be properly controlled.

WHAT TO DO: Monitor phenytoin blood levels and clinical response, and use a higher dose of phenytoin as needed.

179. ↑ **phenytoin (Dilantin)**   **disulfiram (Antabuse)**
        ethotoin (Peganone)
        mephenytoin (Mesantoin)

        Severity: ●●○
Probability: ●●●

USES: Phenytoin is an anticonvulsant drug used for seizure disorders such as epilepsy. Disulfiram is prescribed to deter ingestion of alcoholic beverages.

EFFECT: The effect of phenytoin may be increased.

RESULT: Increased risk of phenytoin toxicity with symptoms such as nystagmus (uncontrolled movement of the eyeballs), double vision, loss of coordination, slurred speech, tremor, lethargy, nausea, vomiting.

WHAT TO DO: Monitor phenytoin blood levels and symptoms, and lower the dose of phenytoin as needed.

180. ↓ **phenytoin (Dilantin)**   **folic acid**
ethotoin (Peganone)
mephenytoin (Mesantoin)

Severity: ●●○
Probability: ●○○

USES: Phenytoin is an anticonvulsant drug used for seizure

disorders such as epilepsy. Folic acid is an essential vitamin found
in liver, yeast, green leafy vegetables, and fruits, and in some vitamin
supplements.
EFFECT: The effect of phenytoin may be decreased.
RESULT: The condition treated with phenytoin may not be properly
controlled.
WHAT TO DO: Monitor phenytoin blood levels and clinical response,
and use a higher dose of phenytoin as needed.

181. ↑ **phenytoin (Dilantin)**   **Isoniazid**
ethotoin (Peganone)   INH, Laniazid, Nydrazid
mephenytoin (Mesantoin)   Rifamate, Rimactane/INH

Severity: ●●○
Probability: ●●●

USES: Phenytoin is an anticonvulsant drug used for seizure disorders
such as epilepsy. Isoniazid is a specialized antibiotic used for tuberculosis.
EFFECT: The effect of phenytoin may be increased.
RESULT: Increased risk of phenytoin toxicity with symptoms such as
nystagmus (uncontrolled movement of the eyeballs), double vision, loss
of coordination, slurred speech, tremor, lethargy, nausea, vomiting.
WHAT TO DO: Monitor phenytoin blood levels and symptoms, and
lower the dose of phenytoin as needed.

182. ↑ **phenytoin (Dilantin)**   **phenacemide**
   (Phenurone)

ethotoin (Peganone)
mephenytoin (Mesantoin)

Severity: ●●○
Probability: ●○○

USES: Phenytoin is an anticonvulsant drug used for seizure disorders such as epilepsy. Phenacemide is an anticonvulsant drug used for severe epilepsy resistant to other drugs.

EFFECT: The effect of phenytoin may be increased.

RESULT: Increased risk of phenytoin toxicity with symptoms such as nystagmus (uncontrolled movement of the eyeballs), double vision, loss of coordination, slurred speech, tremor, lethargy, nausea, vomiting.

WHAT TO DO: Monitor phenytoin blood levels and symptoms, and lower the dose of phenytoin as needed.

183. ↑ phenytoin (Dilantin)   phenylbutazone
                                              (Butazolidin)
       ethotoin (Peganone)   oxyphenbutazone
       mephenytoin (Mesantoin)

       Severity: ●●○
       Probability: ●●○

USES: Phenytoin is an anticonvulsant drug used for seizure disorders such as epilepsy. Phenylbutazone is used for the pain and inflammation of arthritic-type conditions.

EFFECT: The effect of phenytoin may be increased.

RESULT: Increased risk of phenytoin toxicity with symptoms such as nystagmus (uncontrolled movement of the eyeballs), double vision, loss of coordination, slurred speech, tremor, lethargy, nausea, vomiting.

WHAT TO DO: Monitor phenytoin blood levels and symptoms, and lower the dose of phenytoin as needed.

184. ↓ phenytoin (Dilantin)   rifampin
       ethotoin (Peganone)   Rifadin
       mephenytoin (Mesantoin)   Rifamate
                                              Rimactane
                                              Rimactane/INH

       Severity: ●●○
       Probability: ●○○

USES: Phenytoin is an anticonvulsant drug used for seizure disorders such as epilepsy. Rifampin is a specialized antibiotic used for tuberculosis and may also be given to suspected meningitis carriers.

EFFECT: The effect of phenytoin may be decreased.

RESULT: The condition treated with phenytoin may not be properly controlled.

WHAT TO DO: Monitor phenytoin blood levels and clinical response, and use a higher dose of phenytoin as needed.

185. ↓ **phenytoin (Dilantin)**   **sucralfate (Carafate)**
ethotoin (Peganone)
mephenytoin (Mesantoin)

Severity: ●●○
Probability: ●○○

USES: Phenytoin is an anticonvulsant drug used for seizure disorders such as epilepsy. Sucralfate is used for stomach ulcers.

EFFECT: The effect of phenytoin may be decreased.

RESULT: The condition treated with phenytoin may not be properly controlled.

WHAT TO DO: Take the drugs two or more hours apart.

186. ↑ **phenytoin (Dilantin)**   **sulfonamides**
ethotoin (Peganone)   sulfamethizole
mephenytoin (Mesantoin)   Thiosulfil Forte
Urobiotic-250

Severity: ●●○
Probability: ●●○

USES: Phenytoin is an anticonvulsant drug used for seizure disorders such as epilepsy. Sulfamethizole is an antibiotic used for urinary tract infections.

EFFECT: The effect of phenytoin may be increased.

RESULT: Increased risk of phenytoin toxicity with symptoms such as nystagmus (uncontrolled movement of the eyeballs), double vision, loss of coordination, slurred speech, tremor, lethargy, nausea, vomiting.

WHAT TO DO: Monitor phenytoin blood levels and symptoms, and lower the dose of phenytoin as needed.

187. ↑ **phenytoin (Dilantin)**   **trimethoprim**
ethotoin (Peganone)   Bactrim, Proloprim, Septra
mephenytoin (Mesantoin)   Trimpex

  Severity: ●●○
Probability: ●●○

USES: Phenytoin is an anticonvulsant drug used for seizure disorders such as epilepsy. Trimethoprim is an antibiotic used for urinary tract infections.

EFFECT: The effect of phenytoin may be increased.

RESULT: Increased risk of phenytoin toxicity with symptoms such as nystagmus (uncontrolled movement of the eyeballs), double vision, loss of coordination, slurred speech, tremor, lethargy, nausea, vomiting.

WHAT TO DO: Monitor phenytoin blood levels and symptoms, and lower the dose of phenytoin as needed.

188. ↑ **phenytoin (Dilantin)**   ↓ **valproic acid**
                                              (Depakene)

ethotoin (Peganone)
mephenytoin (Mesantoin)

  Severity: ●●○
Probability: ●○○

USES: Phenytoin and valproic acid are anticonvulsant drugs used for seizure disorders such as epilepsy.

EFFECT: The effect of phenytoin may be increased. Also, the effect of valproic acid may be decreased.

RESULT: Increased risk of phenytoin toxicity with symptoms such as nystagmus (uncontrolled movement of the eyeballs), double vision, loss of coordination, slurred speech, tremor, lethargy, nausea vomiting. Also, the condition treated with valproic acid may not be controlled as expected.

WHAT TO DO: Monitor the free serum concentrations of phenytoin and the blood levels of valproic acid. Adjust doses of each drug based on appearance of phenytoin toxicity symptoms or loss of seizure control.

189. ↑ **phenytoin**
ethotoin (Peganone)
mephenytoin (Mesantoin)

↕ **warfarin (Coumadin)**
anisindione (Miradon)
dicumarol

Severity: ●●○
Probability: ●○○

USES: Phenytoin is an anticonvulsant drug used for seizure disorders such as epilepsy. Warfarin is an anticoagulant used to thin the blood and prevent it from clotting.

EFFECT: This is a complex interaction. The effect of phenytoin may be increased. Also, the effect of warfarin may at first be increased, then decreased.

RESULT: Phenytoin—increased risk of toxicity with symptoms such as nystagmus (uncontrolled movement of the eyeballs), double vision, loss of coordination, slurred speech, tremor, lethargy, nausea, vomiting. Warfarin—increased risk of bleeding at first. One to two weeks later, a decreased effect may result in loss of anticoagulant control.

WHAT TO DO: Avoid this combination if feasible. If used, closely monitor phenytoin blood levels and prothrombin times, and observe for clinical response, phenytoin toxicity symptoms, seizure activity, and bleeding.

190. ↓ **piroxicam (Feldene)**

cholestyramine (Questran)

Severity: ●○○
Probability: ●●○

USES: Piroxicam is a nonsteroidal antiinflammatory drug (NSAID) used for pain and inflammation in arthritic-type conditions and for general pain and inflammation. Cholestyramine is used to lower cholesterol blood levels.

EFFECT: The effect of piroxicam may be decreased.

RESULT: The condition treated with piroxicam may not be properly controlled.

WHAT TO DO: Monitor clinical response and use a higher dose of piroxicam as needed.

191.   ↑ **potassium**   **ACE Inhibitors**

foods high in potassium   captopril (Capoten)
potassium acid phosphate   enalapril (Vasotec)
  K-Phos   lisinopril (Prinivil, Zestril)
potassium bicarbonate   ramipril (Altace)
  K-Lyte, Klor-Con/EF
  Klorvess
potassium chloride
  K-Dur, K-Lor, K-Lyte
  K-Norm,K-Tab, Kaochlor
  Kaon Cl, Kay Ciel
  Klor-Con, Klorvess
  Klotrix, Micro-K
  Slow-K, Ten-K
potassium citrate
  Alka-Seltzer, K-Lyte
  Polycitra, Resol, Urocit-K
potassium gluconate
  Kaon, Kolyum
potassium iodide
  Elixophyllin-KI, Iodo-Niacin
  Mudrane, Pediacof, SSKI
potassium phosphate
  K-Phos, Neutra-Phos

Severity: ●●○
Probability: ●○○

USES: Potassium supplementation is used to replace body potassium that is lost due to the use of certain diuretics (called potassium-wasting diuretics). Foods high in potassium: cereals, dried peas and beans, fresh vegetables, fruits, fruit juices, sunflower seeds, watermelon, nuts, molasses, cocoa, fresh fish, beef, ham, poultry. ACE inhibitors are used for high blood pressure and heart failure.

EFFECT: Potassium levels may be increased in certain patients.

RESULT: Possible hyperkalemia (excessive potassium in the blood) with symptoms such as muscular weakness, numbness or paralysis, slow heart beat, heart beat irregularities.

WHAT TO DO: Closely monitor potassium blood levels and symptoms, and adjust the potassium dose as needed.

192. ↑ **potassium**

foods high in potassium
potassium acid phosphate
  K-Phos
potassium bicarbonate
  K-Lyte, Klor-Con/EF
  Klorvess
potassium chloride
  K-Dur, K-Lor, K-Lyte
  K-Norm, K-Tab, Kaochlor
  Kaon Cl, Kay Ciel
  Klor-Con, Klorvess, Klotrix
  Micro-K, Slow-K, Ten-K
potassium citrate
  Alka-Seltzer, K-Lyte
  Polycitra, Resol, Urocit-K
potassium gluconate
  Kaon, Kolyum
potassium iodide
  Elixophyllin-KI, Iodo-Niacin
  Mudrane, Pediacof, SSKI
potassium phosphate
  K-Phos, Neutra-Phos

**diuretics,
potassium-sparing**

amiloride (Midamor)
spironolactone (Aldactone)
triamterene (Dyrenium)

Severity: ●●●
Probability: ●●●

USES: Potassium supplementation is used to replace body potassium that is lost, especially due to the use of certain diuretics (called potassium-wasting diuretics). Foods high in potassium: cereals, dried peas and beans, fresh vegetables, fruits, fruit juices, sunflower seeds, watermelon, nuts, molasses, cocoa, fresh fish, beef, ham, poultry. Diuretics are used to rid the body of excess fluid—this makes them effective in treating congestive heart failure, high blood pressure, cirrhosis of the liver, and kidney dysfunction.

EFFECT: Increased potassium retention by the body.

RESULT: Severe hyperkalemia (excessive potassium in the blood) with symptoms such as muscular weakness, numbness or paralysis, slow or irregular heart beat. Disabilities and deaths have resulted.

WHAT TO DO: Closely monitor potassium blood levels and watch for symptoms. Avoid this combination if possible.

193. ↑ **prazosin (Minipress)**

beta blockers
acebutolol (Sectral)
atenolol (Tenormin)
betaxolol (Kerlone)
carteolol (Cartrol)
esmolol (Brevibloc)
labetalol (Normodyne,
  Trandate)
metoprolol (Lopressor)
nadolol (Corgard)
penbutolol (Levatol)
pindolol (Visken)
propranolol (Inderal)
timolol (Blocadren)

Severity: ●●○
Probability: ●●○

USES: Prazosin is used for high blood pressure. Beta blockers are used for high blood pressure, angina heart pain, and irregular heart beats. Some have other uses, such as in the prevention of migraine headache and to calm the physical manifestations of "stage fright."

EFFECT: The effect of prazosin may be increased.

RESULT: Increased risk of postural hypotension (the blood pressure drops too low upon standing up) with dizziness, faintness.

WHAT TO DO: Be aware of this effect and stand up slowly after sitting or lying.

194. ↑ **prazosin (Minipress)**

verapamil
(Calan, Isoptin)

Severity: ●●○
Probability: ●○○

USES: Prazosin is used for high blood pressure. Verapamil is a calcium channel blocker used for high blood pressure, angina heart pain, and irregular heart beats.

EFFECT: The effect of prazosin may be increased.

RESULT: Increased risk of postural hypotension (the blood pressure drops too low upon standing up) with dizziness and faintness, especially when verapamil is first added to prazosin therapy.

WHAT TO DO: Be aware of this effect and stand up slowly after sitting or lying.

195. ↑**primidone (Mysoline)**   **phenytoin (Dilantin)**
                                                ethotoin (Peganone)
                                                mephenytoin (Mesantoin)

       Severity: ●●○
Probability: ●●○

USES: Both primidone and phenytoin are anticonvulsant drugs used for seizure disorders such as epilepsy.

EFFECT: The conversion of primidone to phenobarbital (one of primidone's normal breakdown products) may be increased.

RESULT: Increased risk of adverse effects from phenobarbital such as drowsiness, dizziness, loss of coordination and alertness.

WHAT TO DO: Monitor blood levels of primidone and phenobarbital, and watch for symptoms.

196.   **probenecid**   **salicylates**
          Benemid, ColBENEMID   aspirin
                                          Alka Seltzer, Anacin
                                          Ascriptin, Aspergum, Bayer
                                          Bufferin, Cama, Ecotrin
                                          Empirin, Measurin,
                                          Momentum, Persistin,
                                          St. Joseph
                                          bismuth subsalicylate
                                          Pepto Bismol
                                          choline salicylate
                                          Arthropan
                                          magnesium salicylate
                                          Doan's
                                          salsalate (Disalcid)
                                          sodium salicylate (Uracel)
                                          sodium thiosalicylate (Tusal)

       Severity: ●●○
Probability: ●●○

USES: Probenecid is used for the hyperuricemia (excess uric acid in the blood) associated with gout and gouty arthritis. Salicylates are primarily used for the pain and inflammation of arthritic-type conditions and for general pain, fever, and inflammation.

EFFECT: The uricosuric (uric acid lowering) effect of both probenecid and salicylates may be decreased.

RESULT: Certain conditions treated may not be properly controlled.

WHAT TO DO: Avoid large doses of salicylates when using proben-ecid. Occasional doses of salicylates in smaller doses may not interact.

197. ↑ **procainamide**   **amiodarone**
                                                      (Cordarone)

Procan, Procan SR
Pronestyl, Pronestyl-SR

Severity: ●●○
Probability: ●●○

USES: Procainamide is used for heart beat irregularities. Amiodarone is recommended only for life-threatening heart beat irregularities of the ventricular type.

EFFECT: The effect of procainamide may be increased.

RESULT: Increased risk of procainamide toxicity with symptoms such as a fall in blood pressure, heart block (disruption in the nerve transmission required for proper heart beat), and a serious heart beat irregularity called ventricular fibrillation.

WHAT TO DO: Monitor procainamide blood levels and symptoms, and lower the dose of procainamide as needed.

198. ↑ **procainamide**   **cimetidine (Tagamet)**
Procan, Procan SR
Pronestyl, Pronestyl-SR

Severity: ●●○
Probability: ●●○

USES: Procainamide is used for heart beat irregularities. Cimetidine is used for gastric and duodenal ulcers.

EFFECT: The effect of procainamide may be increased.

RESULT: Increased risk of procainamide toxicity with symptoms such as a fall in blood pressure, heart block (disruption in the nerve transmission required for proper heart beat), and a serious heart beat irregularity called ventricular fibrillation.

WHAT TO DO: Monitor procainamide blood levels and symptoms, and lower the dose of procainamide as needed. Avoid this combination if feasible.

199. ↑**procainamide**
 Procan, Procan SR
 Pronestyl, Pronestyl-SR

trimethoprim
Bactrim, Proloprim, Septra
Trimpex

Severity: ●●○
Probability: ●○○

USES: Procainamide is used for heart beat irregularities. Trimethoprim is an antibiotic used for urinary tract infections.

EFFECT: The effect of procainamide may be increased.

RESULT: Increased risk of procainamide toxicity with symptoms such as a fall in blood pressure, heart block (disruption in the nerve transmission required for proper heart beat), and a serious heart beat irregularity called ventricular fibrillation.

WHAT TO DO: Monitor procainamide blood levels and symptoms, and lower the dose of procainamide as needed.

200. ↑**quinidine**

 Cardioquin
 Cin-Quin
 Duraquin
 Quinaglute Dura-Tabs
 Quinalan
 Quinidex Extentabs
 Quinora

**amiodarone
(Cordarone)**

Severity: ●●●
Probability: ●●○

USES: Quinidine is used for heart beat irregularities. Amiodarone is recommended only for life-threatening heart beat irregularities of the ventricular type.

EFFECT: The effect of quinidine may be increased.

RESULT: Increased risk of quinidine toxicity with symptoms such as vertigo, fall in blood pressure, heart block (disruption in the nerve transmission required for proper heart beat), and a serious heart beat irregularity called ventricular fibrillation.

WHAT TO DO: Monitor quinidine blood levels and symptoms, and lower the dose of quinidine as needed.

201. ↑ **quinidine**
Cardioquin
Cin-Quin
Duraquin
Quinaglute Dura-Tabs
Quinalan
Quinidex Extentabs
Quinora

antacids
AlternaGEL, Amphojel
Camalox, Chooz, Delcid
Di-Gel, Gaviscon, Gelusil
Kudrox, Maalox, Mylanta
Riopan, Rolaids
Titralac, Tums

Severity: ●●○
Probability: ●○○

USES: Quinidine is used for heart beat irregularities. Antacids are used for stomach problems associated with too much stomach acid.

EFFECT: The effect of quinidine may be increased.

RESULT: Increased risk of quinidine toxicity with symptoms such as vertigo, fall in blood pressure, heart block (disruption in the nerve transmission required for proper heart beat), and a serious heart beat irregularity called ventricular fibrillation.

WHAT TO DO: Monitor quinidine blood levels and symptoms, and lower the dose of quinidine as needed. (An aluminum-only antacid such as AlternaGEL, Aludrox, and Amphojel may not interact.)

202. ↓ **quinidine**
Cardioquin
Cin-Quin
Duraquin
Quinaglute Dura-Tabs
Quinalan
Quinidex Extentabs
Quinora

barbiturates
amobarbital (Amytal)
aprobarbital (Alurate)
butabarbital (Butisol)
butalbital
mephobarbital (Mebaral)
pentobarbital (Nembutal)
phenobarbital
primidone (Mysoline)
secobarbital (Seconal)
talbutal (Lotusate)

Severity: ●●○
Probability: ●●○

USES: Quinidine is used for heart beat irregularities. Barbiturates are used as sedatives or sleep inducers; phenobarbital and primidone are used for seizure disorders such as epilepsy.

EFFECT: The effect of quinidine may be decreased.

RESULT: The condition treated with quinidine may not be properly controlled.

WHAT TO DO: Monitor quinidine blood levels and clinical response, and use a higher dose of quinidine as needed.

203. ↑ **quinidine**   **cimetidine (Tagamet)**
Cardioquin
Cin-Quin
Duraquin
Quinaglute Dura-Tabs
Quinalan
Quinidex Extentabs
Quinora

Severity: ●●○
Probability: ●○○

USES: Quinidine is used for heart beat irregularities. Cimetidine is used for gastric and duodenal ulcers.

EFFECT: The effect of quinidine may be increased.

RESULT: Increased risk of quinidine toxicity with symptoms such as vertigo, fall in blood pressure, heart block (disruption in the nerve transmission required for proper heart beat), and a serious heart beat irregularity called ventricular fibrillation.

WHAT TO DO: Monitor quinidine blood levels and symptoms, and lower the dose of quinidine as needed. Avoid this combination if feasible.

204. ↓ **quinidine**   **phenytoin (Dilantin)**
Cardioquin
Cin-Quin
Duraquin
Quinaglute Dura-Tabs
Quinalan
Quinidex Extentabs
Quinora

Severity: ●●○
Probability: ●○○

USES: Quinidine is used for heart beat irregularities. Phenytoin is an anticonvulsant drug used for seizure disorders such as epilepsy.

EFFECT: The effect of quinidine may be decreased.

RESULT: The condition treated with quinidine may not be properly controlled.

WHAT TO DO: Monitor quinidine blood levels and clinical response, and use a higher dose of quinidine as needed. Avoid this combination if feasible.

205. ↓ **quinidine**   **rifampin**
Cardioquin   Rifadin
Cin-Quin   Rifamate
Duraquin   Rimactane
Quinaglute Dura-Tabs   Rimactane/INH
Quinalan
Quinidex Extentabs
Quinora

Severity: ●●○
Probability: ●●○

USES: Quinidine is used for heart beat irregularities. Rifampin is a specialized antibiotic used for tuberculosis and may also be given to suspected meningitis carriers.

EFFECT: The effect of quinidine may be decreased.

RESULT: The condition treated with quinidine may not be properly controlled.

WHAT TO DO: Monitor quinidine blood levels and clinical response, and use a higher dose of quinidine as needed.

206. ↑ **salicylates**   **alcohol (ethanol)**
aspirin   beer, liquor, wine
Alka Seltzer, Anacin,
Ascriptin, Aspergum, Bayer
Bufferin, Cama, Ecotrin
Empirin, Measurin, Momentum
Persistin, St. Joseph

Severity: ●○○
Probability: ●○○

USES: Aspirin is used for the pain and inflammation of arthritic-type conditions and for general pain, fever, and inflammation.

EFFECT: The blood-thinning effect of aspirin may be increased.

RESULT: Increased risk of adverse effects such as bleeding and blood loss from the GI (gastrointestinal) tract.

WHAT TO DO: Moderate alcohol intake or taking aspirin 12 or more hours after alcohol intake minimizes risk. Also, GI blood loss is decreased by using an enteric-coated tablet (e.g., Ecotrin), an extended-release product (e.g., Bayer 8-Hour, Measurin, ZORprin), or a buffered aspirin-containing solution (e.g., Alka-Seltzer).

207. ↓ **salicylates**
aspirin
Alka Seltzer, Anacin
Ascriptin, Aspergum, Bayer
Bufferin, Cama, Ecotrin
Empirin, Measurin
Momentum, Persistin
St. Joseph
bismuth subsalicylate
Pepto Bismol
choline salicylate
Arthropan
magnesium salicylate
Doan's
salsalate (Disalcid)
sodium salicylate (Uracel)
sodium thiosalicylate (Tusal)

antacids
AlternaGEL, Amphojel
Camalox, Chooz, Delcid
Di-Gel, Gaviscon, Gelusil
Kudrox, Maalox, Mylanta
Riopan, Rolaids
Titralac, Tums

Severity: ●○○
Probability: ●●○

USES: Salicylates are used for the pain and inflammation of arthritic-type conditions and for general pain, fever, and inflammation. Antacids are used for stomach problems associated with too much stomach acid.

EFFECT: The effect of the salicylate may be decreased.

RESULT: The condition treated with the salicylate may not be properly controlled.

WHAT TO DO: Monitor the clinical response and use a higher dose of the salicylate as needed.

208. ↑ **salicylates**

aspirin
  Alka Seltzer, Anacin
  Ascriptin, Aspergum, Bayer
  Bufferin, Cama, Ecotrin
  Empirin, Measurin
  Momentum, Persistin
  St. Joseph
bismuth subsalicylate
  Pepto Bismol
choline salicylate
  Arthropan
magnesium salicylate
  Doan's
salsalate (Disalcid)
sodium salicylate (Uracel)
sodium thiosalicylate (Tusal)

↑ **carbonic anhydrase inhibitors**

acetazolamide (Diamox)
dichlorphenamide (Daranide)
methazolamide (Neptazane)

Severity: ●●○
Probability: ●○○

USES: Salicylates are used for the pain and inflammation of arthritic-type conditions and for general pain, fever, and inflammation. Carbonic anhydrase inhibitors are a specialized type of diuretic used for glaucoma (increased pressure within the eye).

EFFECT: The effect of both drugs may be increased.

RESULT: Increased risk of aspirin toxicity with symptoms such as confusion, drowsiness, lethargy, hyperventilation, appetite loss, tinnitus (ringing in the ears). Also, increased risk of carbonic anhydrase inhibitor-induced metabolic acidosis with symptoms such as nausea and vomiting, diarrhea, headache, altered levels of consciousness, tremors, convulsions.

WHAT TO DO: Monitor salicylate blood levels and acid base balance, and watch for symptoms. Avoid this combination if feasible.

209. ↓ **salicylates**

aspirin
  Alka Seltzer, Anacin
  Ascriptin, Aspergum, Bayer
  Bufferin, Cama, Ecotrin
  Empirin, Measurin

corticosteroids

betamethasone (Celestone)
cortisone (Cortone)
dexamethasone (Decadron)
fludrocortisone (Florinef)
hydrocortisone (Cortef)

Momentum, Persistin
St. Joseph
bismuth subsalicylate
Pepto Bismol
choline salicylate
Arthropan
magnesium salicylate
Doan's
salsalate (Disalcid)
sodium salicylate (Uracel)
sodium thiosalicylate (Tusal)

methylprednisolone (Medrol)
prednisolone (Delta-Cortef)
prednisone (Deltasone)
triamcinolone (Aristocort)

Severity: ●●○
Probability: ●●○

USES: Salicylates are used for the pain and inflammation of arthritic-type conditions and for general pain, fever, and inflammation. Corticosteroids are used for a wide spectrum of conditions, including arthritis, allergies, and asthma.

EFFECT: The effect of the salicylate may be decreased.

RESULT: The condition treated with the salicylate may not be properly controlled.

WHAT TO DO: Monitor salicylate blood levels and clinical response, and use a higher dose of the salicylate as needed.

---

210. ↓ **salicylates**
aspirin
Alka Seltzer, Anacin
Ascriptin, Aspergum, Bayer
Bufferin, Cama, Ecotrin
Empirin, Measurin
Momentum, Persistin
St. Joseph
bismuth subsalicylate
Pepto Bismol
choline salicylate
Arthropan
magnesium salicylate
Doan's
salsalate (Disalcid)
sodium salicylate (Uracel)

urinary alkalinizers
potassium citrate
Alka-Seltzer
K-Lyte
sodium acetate
sodium bicarbonate
Alka-Seltzer
Citrocarbonate
sodium citrate
Alka-Seltzer
sodium lactate
tromethamine

Severity: ●○○
Probability: ●●●

USES: Salicylates are used for the pain and inflammation of arthritic-type conditions and for general pain, fever, and inflammation. Urinary alkalinizers are used in some antacids and in some potassium supplement products.

EFFECT: The effect of the salicylate may be decreased.

RESULT: The condition treated with the salicylate may not be properly controlled.

WHAT TO DO: Monitor salicylate blood levels and clinical response, and use a higher dose of the salicylate as needed. (The patient may also use home pH tests to monitor urine acidity; the higher the pH (the less acidic), the more the decrease in the salicylate effect.)

211.   **smoking (e.g., cigarette)** ↓ **antidepressants, tricylic**
amitriptyline
  Elavil, Endep
amoxapine (Asendin)
clomipramine (Anafranil)
desipramine
  Norpramin, Pertofrane
doxepin (Adapin, Sinequan)
imipramine (Tofranil)
nortriptyline
  Aventyl, Pamelor
protriptyline (Vivactil)
trimipramine (Surmontil)

Severity: ●○○
Probability: ●○○

USES: Antidepressants are used for clinical depression.

EFFECT: The effect of the antidepressant may be decreased.

RESULT: The condition treated with the antidepressant may not be properly controlled.

WHAT TO DO: Monitor the clinical response and adjust the dose of the antidepressant as warranted.

212. **smoking (e.g., cigarette)** ↓ **benzodiazepines**

alprazolam (Xanax)
chlordiazepoxide (Librium)
clonazepam (Klonopin)
clorazepate (Tranxene)
diazepam (Valium)
estazolam (ProSam)
flurazepam (Dalmane)
halazepam (Paxipam)
lorazepam (Ativan)
midazolam (Versed)
oxazepam (Serax)
prazepam (Centrax)
quazepam (Doral)
temazepam (Restoril)
triazolam (Halcion)

Severity: ●○○
Probability: ●○○

USES: Benzodiazepines are used for anxiety; some are used to induce sleep.

EFFECT: The effect of the benzodiazepine may be decreased. (This effect seems to be directly proportional to the number of cigarettes smoked per day.)

RESULT: The condition treated with the benzodiazepine may not be properly controlled.

WHAT TO DO: Monitor the clinical response and use a higher dose of the benzodiazepine as needed.

213. **smoking (e.g., cigarette)** **birth control pills**

Brevicon, Demulen, Genora
Levlen, Lo-Ovral, Loestrin
Modicon, Nelova, Norcept
Nordette, Norethin, Norinyl
Norlestrin, Ortho-Novum
Ovcon, Ovral, Tri-Levlen
Tri-Norinyl

Severity: ●●○
Probability: ●●○

USES: Birth control pills are used to prevent pregnancy.

RESULT: Increased risk of birth control pill-induced adverse cardio-vascular effects such as heart attack and blood clot formation. The risk is greater in people over age 35 and in those smoking more than 15 cigarettes a day.

WHAT TO DO: Do not smoke; if you do smoke, consider using an alternative to the birth control pill.

214.   smoking (e.g., cigarette)   estrogens
chlorotrianisene (Tace)
conjugated estrogens
 Premarin
diethylstilbestrol (DES)
esterified estrogens
 Estratab, Menest
estradiol (Estrace)
estropipate (Ogen)
ethinyl estradiol
 Estinyl, Feminone
mestranol (Enovid)
quinestrol (Estrovis)

Severity: ●●○
Probability: ●●○

USES: Estrogens are used for the symptoms of menopause and for osteoporosis, and also have other uses.

RESULT: Increased risk of estrogen-induced adverse cardiovascular effects such as heart attack and blood clot formation. The risk is greater in people over age 35 and in those smoking more than 15 cigarettes a day.

WHAT TO DO: Do not smoke.

215.   smoking (e.g., cigarette)   insulin

Severity: ●○○
Probability: ●●○

USES: Insulin is used for diabetes.

EFFECT: The effect of insulin may be decreased. (Diabetics who smoke heavily may require up to one-third more insulin than non-smoking diabetics.)

RESULT: Diabetes may not be properly controlled.

WHAT TO DO: Do not smoke. If you do smoke, be aware that a change in the number of cigarettes smoked a day may change insulin requirements.

216.   **smoking (e.g., cigarette)** ↓ **pentazocine (Talwin)**

     Severity: ●○○
Probability: ●○○

USES: Pentazocine is a narcotic pain reliever.

EFFECT: The effect of pentazocine may be decreased.

RESULT: The condition treated with pentazocine may not be properly controlled.

WHAT TO DO: Monitor the clinical response and use a higher dose of pentazocine as needed. Option: use an alternative to pentazocine.

217.   **smoking (e.g., cigarette)** ↓ **phenothiazines**
            acetophenazine (Tindal)
            chlorpromazine (Thorazine)
            fluphenazine (Permitil,
              Prolixin)
            mesoridazine (Serentil)
            perphenazine (Trilafon)
            prochlorperazine (Compazine)
            promazine (Sparine)
            promethazine (Phenergan)
            thioridazine (Mellaril)
            trifluoperazine (Stelazine)

     Severity: ●○○
Probability: ●○○

USES: Phenothiazines are antipsychotic drugs used for brain disorders such as schizophrenia, paranoia, and manic-depressive illness.

EFFECT: The effect of the phenothiazine may be decreased. (This effect seems to be directly proportional to the number of cigarettes smoked per day.)

RESULT: The condition treated with the phenothiazine may not be properly controlled.

WHAT TO DO: Monitor the clinical response and use a higher dose of the phenothiazine as needed.

218.   smoking (e.g., cigarette) ↓ **propoxyphene**
Darvon, Dolene, Wygesic
Darvocet-N

Severity: ●○○
Probability: ●○○

USES: Propoxyphene is a pain reliever.

EFFECT: The effect of propoxyphene may be decreased. (This effect seems to be directly proportional to the number of cigarettes smoked per day.)

RESULT: The condition treated with propoxyphene may not be properly controlled.

WHAT TO DO: Monitor the clinical response and use a higher dose of propoxyphene as needed. Option: use an alternative to propoxyphene.

219.   smoking (e.g., cigarette) ↓ **theophyllines**
aminophylline
  Somophyllin
dyphylline
  Dilor, Lufyllin
theophylline
  Aerolate, Bronkodyl
  Bronkaid, Constant-T
  Elixophyllin, Marax
  Mudrane, Primatene
  Quibron, Respbid
  Slo-bid, Slo-Phyllin
  T-PHYL, Tedral, Theo-24
  Theo-dur, Theo-Organidin
  Theobid, Theolair
  Theospan-SR, Theostat 80
  Uniphyl

Severity: ●○○
Probability: ●●○

USES: Theophyllines are used for asthma and for bronchospasm associated with chronic bronchitis and emphysema.

EFFECT: The effect of theophylline may be decreased. (When smoking is stopped, this effect dissipates slowly over a period of several months.)

RESULT: The condition treated with theophylline may not be properly controlled.

WHAT TO DO: Monitor the clinical response and adjust the dose of theophylline as needed.

220. ↓ sodium polystyrene sulfonate

Kayexalate

antacids

AlternaGEL, Amphojel
Camalox, Chooz, Delcid
Di-Gel, Gaviscon, Gelusil
Kudrox, Maalox
milk of magnesia, Mylanta
Riopan, Rolaids
Titralac, Tums

Severity: ●●○
Probability: ●●●

USES: Sodium polystyrene sulfonate is used for hyperkalemia (excessive potassium in the blood). Antacids are used for stomach disorders associated with too much acid; milk of magnesia is used as a laxative.

EFFECT: The effect of sodium polystyrene sulfonate may be decreased; in addition, metabolic alkalosis (excessive alkalinity—as opposed to acidity—of body fluids) may occur.

RESULT: The condition treated with sodium polystyrene sulfonate may not be properly controlled; also, adverse effects from metabolic alkalosis such as apathy, irritability, delirium, dehydration, involuntary muscular contractions.

WHAT TO DO: Take the two drugs several hours apart.

221. ↓ spironolactone (Aldactone)

salicylates

aspirin
Alka Seltzer, Anacin
Ascriptin, Aspergum, Bayer
Bufferin, Cama, Ecotrin
Empirin, Measurin
Momentum, Persistin
St. Joseph
bismuth subsalicylate

Pepto Bismol
choline salicylate (Arthropan)
magnesium salicylate
 Doan's
salsalate (Disalcid)
sodium salicylate (Uracel)
sodium thiosalicylate (Tusal)

Severity: ●○○
Probability: ●○○

USES: Spironolactone is a potassium-sparing diuretic used to rid the body of excess fluid—this makes it effective in treating congestive heart failure, high blood pressure, cirrhosis of the liver, kidney dysfunction, and hypokalemia (low blood levels of potassium); it is also used for hyperaldosteronism (excessive production of the hormone aldosterone by the adrenal gland). Salicylates are used for pain, fever, and inflammation.

EFFECT: The effect of spironolactone may be decreased.

RESULT: The condition treated with spironolactone may not be properly controlled.

WHAT TO DO: Monitor blood pressure and sodium blood levels, and use a higher dose of spironolactone as needed.

222. ↓ **sulfinpyrazone   salicylates**
        (Anturane)

aspirin
 Alka Seltzer, Anacin
 Ascriptin, Aspergum, Bayer
 Bufferin, Cama, Ecotrin
 Empirin, Measurin
 Momentum, Persistin
 St. Joseph
bismuth subsalicylate
 Pepto Bismol
choline salicylate (Arthropan)
magnesium salicylate
 Doan's
salsalate (Disalcid)
sodium salicylate (Uracel)
sodium thiosalicylate (Tusal)

Severity: ●●○
Probability: ●●●

USES: Sulfinpyrazone is used for the hyperuricemia (excess uric acid in the blood) associated with gouty arthritis. Salicylates are primarily used for the pain and inflammation of arthritic-type conditions and for general pain, fever, and inflammation.

EFFECT: The uricosuric (uric acid-lowering) effect of sulfinpyrazone may be decreased.

RESULT: The condition treated with sulfinpyrazone may not be properly controlled.

WHAT TO DO: Avoid using more than occasional small doses of salicylates during sulfinpyrazone therapy.

223. **sulfonylureas** **alcohol (ethanol)**
    acetohexamide (Dymelor)   beer, liquor, wine
    chlorpropamide (Diabinese)
    glipizide (Glucotrol)
    glyburide (Diabeta,
      Micronase)
    tolazamide (Tolinase)
    tolbutamide (Orinase)

Severity: ●●○
Probability: ●●●

USES: Sulfonylureas are used to lower blood sugar in diabetes therapy.

RESULT: Increased risk of altered blood sugar control, especially hypoglycemia (low blood sugar); also, a disulfiram-type reaction (flushing, nausea, vomiting, dizziness, shortness of breath, severe headache, visual disturbances, heart palpitations, possible unconsciousness) may occur.

WHAT TO DO: Avoid drinking too much alcohol. Smaller amounts, especially if taken with a meal, may not interact significantly.

224. ↑ **sulfonylureas** **chloramphenicol**
    acetohexamide (Dymelor)   Chloromycetin
    chlorpropamide (Diabinese)
    glipizide (Glucotrol)
    glyburide (Diabeta,
      Micronase)
    tolazamide (Tolinase)
    tolbutamide (Orinase)

Severity: ●●○
Probability: ●○○

USES: Sulfonylureas are used to lower blood sugar in diabetes therapy. Chloramphenicol is an antibiotic used for microbial infections.

EFFECT: The effect of the sulfonylurea may be increased.

RESULT: Increased risk of hypoglycemia (low blood sugar) with symptoms such as nervousness, faintness, weakness, sweating, confusion, heart beat irregularities, rapid heart beats, loss of coordination, visual disturbances.

WHAT TO DO: Monitor glucose blood levels and watch for adverse symptoms. Lower the dose of the sulfonylurea as needed.

225. ⬆ **sulfonylureas**   **clofibrate (Atromid-S)**
  acetohexamide (Dymelor)
  chlorpropamide (Diabinese)
  glipizide (Glucotrol)
  glyburide (Diabeta,
      Micronase)
  tolazamide (Tolinase)
  tolbutamide (Orinase)

Severity: ●○○
Probability: ●○○

USES: Sulfonylureas are used to lower blood sugar in diabetes therapy. Clofibrate is used to lower high blood levels of cholesterol and/or triglycerides.

EFFECT: The effect of the sulfonylurea may be increased.

RESULT: Increased risk of hypoglycemia (low blood sugar) with symptoms such as nervousness, faintness, weakness, sweating, confusion, heart beat irregularities, rapid heart beats, loss of coordination, visual disturbances.

WHAT TO DO: Monitor blood glucose levels and watch for adverse symptoms. Lower the dose of the sulfonylurea as needed.

226. ⬇ **sulfonylureas**   **diuretics, thiazide**
  acetohexamide (Dymelor)   bendroflumethiazide
  chlorpropamide (Diabinese)   Naturetin
                      benzthiazide (Aquatag)

glipizide (Glucotrol)
glyburide (Diabeta, Micronase)
tolazamide (Tolinase)
tolbutamide (Orinase)

chlorothiazide (Diuril)
chlorthalidone (Hygroton)
cyclothiazide (Anhydron)
hydrochlorothiazide
  Esidrix, HydroDiuril
hydroflumethiazide (Saluron)
indapamide (Lozol)
  methyclothiazide (Enduron)
metolazone (Diulo,
  Zaroxolyn)
polythiazide (Renese)
quinethazone (Hydromox)
trichlormethiazide (Naqua)

Severity: ●●○
Probability: ●●○

USES: Sulfonylureas are used to lower blood sugar in diabetes therapy. Diuretics are used to rid the body of excess fluid—this makes them effective in treating congestive heart failure, high blood pressure, cirrhosis of the liver, and kidney dysfunction.

EFFECT: The effect of the sulfonylurea may be decreased. (This effect may not appear for several days or months.)

RESULT: The condition treated with the sulfonylurea may not be properly controlled.

WHAT TO DO: Monitor blood glucose levels and use a higher dose of the sulfonylurea as needed.

227. ↑ **sulfonylureas**   **fenfluramine (Pondimin)**
acetohexamide (Dymelor)
chlorpropamide (Diabinese)
glipizide (Glucotrol)
glyburide (Diabeta,
    Micronase)
tolazamide (Tolinase)
tolbutamide (Orinase)

Severity: ●○○
Probability: ●○○

USES: Sulfonylureas are used to lower blood sugar in diabetes therapy. Fenfluramine is an appetite suppressant used in short term therapy for weight loss.

EFFECT: The effect of the sulfonylurea may be increased.

RESULT: Increased risk of hypoglycemia (low blood sugar) with symptoms such as nervousness, faintness, weakness, sweating, confusion, heart beat irregularities, rapid heart beats, loss of coordination, visual disturbances.

WHAT TO DO: Monitor blood glucose levels and watch for adverse symptoms. Lower the dose of the sulfonylurea as needed.

228. ↑ **sulfonylureas**   **MAO inhibitors**
    acetohexamide (Dymelor)   isocarboxazid (Marplan)
    chlorpropamide (Diabinese)   pargyline (Eutonyl)
    glipizide (Glucotrol)   phenelzine (Nardil)
    glyburide (Diabeta,   tranylcypromine
       Micronase)   Parnate
    tolazamide (Tolinase)
    tolbutamide (Orinase)

     Severity: ●●○
Probability: ●○○

USES: Sulfonylureas are used to lower blood sugar in diabetes therapy. MAO inhibitors are used for some cases of clinical depression.

EFFECT: The effect of the sulfonylurea may be increased.

RESULT: Increased risk of hypoglycemia (low blood sugar) with symptoms such as nervousness, faintness, weakness, sweating, confusion, heart beat irregularities, rapid heart beats, loss of coordination, visual disturbances.

WHAT TO DO: Monitor blood glucose levels and watch for adverse symptoms. Lower the dose of the sulfonylurea as needed.

229. ↑ **sulfonylureas**   **phenylbutazone**
                                       (Butazolidin)
    acetohexamide (Dymelor)
    chlorpropamide (Diabinese)
    glipizide (Glucotrol)
    glyburide (Diabeta,
       Micronase)
    tolazamide (Tolinase)
    tolbutamide (Orinase)

Severity: ●●○
Probability: ●●●

USES: Sulfonylureas are used to lower blood sugar in diabetes therapy. Phenylbutazone is used for the pain and inflammation of arthritic-type conditions.

EFFECT: The effect of the sulfonylurea may be increased.

RESULT: Increased risk of hypoglycemia (low blood sugar) with symptoms such as nervousness, faintness, weakness, sweating, confusion, heart beat irregularities, rapid heart beats, loss of coordination, visual disturbances.

WHAT TO DO: Monitor blood glucose levels and watch for adverse symptoms. Lower the dose of the sulfonylurea as needed. Option: use an alternative to phenylbutazone.

230. ↓ **sulfonylureas**   **rifampin**
       acetohexamide (Dymelor)   Rifadin
       chlorpropamide (Diabinese)   Rifamate
       glipizide (Glucotrol)   Rimactane
       glyburide (Diabeta,   Rimactane/INH
           Micronase)
       tolazamide (Tolinase)
       tolbutamide (Orinase)

Severity: ●●○
Probability: ●○○

USES: Sulfonylureas are used to lower blood sugar in diabetes therapy. Rifampin is a specialized antibiotic used for tuberculosis and may also be given to suspected meningitis carriers.

EFFECT: The effect of the sulfonylurea may be decreased.

RESULT: The condition treated with the sulfonylurea may not be properly controlled.

WHAT TO DO: Monitor blood glucose levels and use a higher dose of the sulfonylurea as needed.

231. ↑ **sulfonylureas**   **salicylates**
       acetohexamide (Dymelor)   aspirin
       chlorpropamide (Diabinese)   Alka Seltzer, Anacin
       glipizide (Glucotrol)   Ascriptin, Aspergum, Bayer
       glyburide (Diabeta, Micronase) Bufferin, Cama, Ecotrin

tolazamide (Tolinase)   Empirin, Measurin,
tolbutamide (Orinase)   Momentum
                                   Persistin, St. Joseph
                                   bismuth subsalicylate
                                    Pepto Bismol
                                   choline salicylate (Arthropan)
                                   magnesium salicylate
                                    Doan's
                                   salsalate (Disalcid)
                                   sodium salicylate (Uracel)
                                   sodium thiosalicylate (Tusal)

Severity: ●●○
Probability: ●●○

USES: Sulfonylureas are used to lower blood sugar in diabetes therapy. Salicylates are primarily used for the pain and inflammation of arthritic-type conditions and for general pain, fever, and inflammation.

EFFECT: The effect of the sulfonylurea may be increased.

RESULT: Increased risk of hypoglycemia (low blood sugar) with symptoms such as nervousness, faintness, weakness, sweating, confusion, heart beat irregularities, rapid heart beats, loss of coordination, visual disturbances.

WHAT TO DO: Monitor blood glucose levels and watch for adverse symptoms. Lower the dose of the sulfonylurea as needed.

232. ↑ **sulfonylureas**   **sulfinpyrazone**
                                        (Anturane)

tolbutamide (Orinase)

Severity: ●●○
Probability: ●○○

USES: Tolbutamide is used to lower blood sugar in diabetes therapy. Sulfinpyrazone is used for the hyperuricemia (excess uric acid in the blood) associated with gouty arthritis.

EFFECT: The effect of tolbutamide may be increased. (It is not known if this interaction occurs with other sulfonylureas.)

RESULT: Increased risk of hypoglycemia (low blood sugar) with symptoms such as nervousness, faintness, weakness, sweating, confusion, heart beat irregularities, rapid heart beats, loss of coordination, visual disturbances.

WHAT TO DO: Monitor blood glucose levels and watch for adverse symptoms. Lower the dose of tolbutamide as needed.

233. ↑ **sulfonylureas**
acetohexamide (Dymelor)
chlorpropamide (Diabinese)
glipizide (Glucotrol)
glyburide (Diabeta,
  Micronase)
tolazamide (Tolinase)
tolbutamide (Orinase)

sulfonamides
sulfadiazine (Microsulfon)
sulfamethizole
  Thiosulfil Forte
sulfamethoxazole (Gantanol)
sulfasalazine (Azulfidine)
sulfisoxazole
  Gantrisin
  Lipo Gantrisin
sulfonamides, multiple
  Triple Sulfa, Neotrizine
  Terfonyl

Severity: ●●○
Probability: ●○○

USES: Sulfonylureas are used to lower blood sugar in diabetes therapy. Sulfonamides are used for urinary tract infections and a variety of other microbial infections.

EFFECT: The effect of the sulfonylurea may be increased.

RESULT: Increased risk of hypoglycemia (low blood sugar) with symptoms such as nervousness, faintness, weakness, sweating, confusion, heart beat irregularities, rapid heart beats, loss of coordination, visual disturbances.

WHAT TO DO: Monitor blood glucose levels and watch for adverse symptoms. Lower the dose of the sulfonylurea as needed. (The sulfonylurea glyburide may not interact.)

234. ↑ **sulfonylureas**
chlorpropamide (Diabinese)

urinary acidifiers
ammonium chloride
  Ipsatol Expectorant Syrup
  P-V-Tussin Syrup
  Quelidrine Syrup
potassium acid phosphate
  K-Phos
  K-Phos No. 2
  Thiacide

sodium acid phosphate
K-Phos No. 2
Uroqid-Acid
Uroqid-Acid No. 2

Severity: ●○○
Probability: ●○○

USES: Sulfonylureas are used to lower blood sugar in diabetes therapy. Urinary acidifiers: ammonium chloride is an expectorant (agent which liquefies mucus) and is used in some cough syrups; potassium acid phosphate and sodium acid phosphate are used to make the urine more acidic.

EFFECT: The effect of chlorpropamide may be increased. (It is not known whether other sulfonylureas interact.)

RESULT: Increased risk of hypoglycemia (low blood sugar) with symptoms such as nervousness, faintness, weakness, sweating, confusion, heart beat irregularities, rapid heart beats, loss of coordination, visual disturbances.

WHAT TO DO: Monitor blood glucose levels and watch for adverse symptoms. Lower the dose of chlorpropamide as needed.

235. ↓ **sulfonylureas**   **urinary alkalinizers**
       chlorpropamide (Diabinese)   potassium citrate
                                                     Alka-Seltzer
                                                     K-Lyte
                                                 sodium acetate
                                                 sodium bicarbonate
                                                     Alka-Seltzer
                                                     Citrocarbonate
                                                 sodium citrate
                                                     Alka-Seltzer
                                                 sodium lactate
                                                 tromethamine

Severity: ●●○
Probability: ●○○

USES: Sulfonylureas are used to lower blood sugar in diabetes therapy. Urinary alkalinizers are used in some antacids and in some potassium supplement products.

EFFECT: The effect of chlorpropamide may be decreased. (It is not known whether other sulfonylureas interact.)

RESULT: The condition treated with chlorpropamide may not be properly controlled.

WHAT TO DO: Monitor blood glucose levels and use a higher dose of chlorpropamide as needed.

236.	↑ **sympathomimetics**	**antidepressants, tricyclic**

↑ **sympathomimetics**
Direct-acting
  dobutamine
  epinephrine
  methoxamine
  norepinephrine
  *phenylephrine

antidepressants, tricyclic
amitriptyline (Elavil, Endep)
amoxapine (Asendin)
clomipramine (Anafranil)
desipramine
  Norpramin, Pertofrane
doxepin (Adapin, Sinequan)
imipramine (Tofranil)
nortriptyline
  Aventyl, Pamelor
protriptyline (Vivactil)
trimipramine (Surmontil)

Severity: ●●○
Probability: ●●●

USES: Sympathomimetics are used to treat shock; phenylephrine is used in nonprescription nasal decongestant sprays and drops (read product labels). Antidepressants are used for clinical depression.

EFFECT: The effect of direct-acting sympathomimetics may be increased.

RESULT: Increased risk of adverse effects such as heart beat irregularities, dangerous rise in blood pressure, headache, fever, visual disturbances.

WHAT TO DO: Watch for symptoms and lower the dose of the sympathomimetic as needed.

237. ↑ **sympathomimetics**   **furazolidone (Furoxone)**
Mixed or indirect-acting
  dopamine
  *ephedrine
  mephentermine
  metaraminol
  *phenylpropanolamine
  *pseudoephedrine

Severity: ●●●
Probability: ●○○

USES: Sympathomimetics are used to treat shock; those marked with an asterisk are used in nonprescription cold and appetite suppressant products (read labels). Furazolidone is used for bacterial and protozoal diarrhea and enteritis (inflammation of the intestines).

EFFECT: The effect of mixed or indirect-acting sympathomimetics may be increased.

RESULT: Increased risk of adverse effects such as heart beat irregularities, dangerous rise in blood pressure, headache, fever, visual disturbances.

WHAT TO DO: Monitor carefully for adverse symptoms. It may be best to avoid this combination.

---

238.   **sympathomimetics**   **MAO inhibitors**

  ↑ Direct-acting   isocarboxazid (Marplan)
   dobutamine   pargyline (Eutonyl)
   epinephrine   phenelzine (Nardil)
   methoxamine   tranylcypromine (Parnate)
   norepinephrine
  ↑ *phenylephrine
  ↑ Mixed or indirect-acting
   dopamine
   *ephedrine
   mephentermine
   metaraminol
   *phenylpropanolamine
   *pseudoephedrine

   Severity: ●●●
Probability: ●●●

USES: Sympathomimetics are used to treat shock; those marked with an asterisk are used in nonprescription cold and appetite suppressant products (read labels). MAO inhibitors are used for some cases of clinical depression.

EFFECT: The effect of mixed or indirect-acting sympathomimetics may be increased markedly. The effect of some direct-acting sympathomimetics may be increased somewhat.

RESULT: Increased risk of adverse effects such as heart beat irregularities, dangerous rise in blood pressure, headache, fever, visual disturbances.

WHAT TO DO: Avoid this potentially dangerous combination.

239. ↑ **sympathomimetics**
     Direct-acting
       dobutamine
       epinephrine
       methoxamine
       Norepinephrine
       *phenylephrine
     Mixed or indirect-acting
       dopamine
       *ephedrine
       mephentermine
       metaraminol
       *phenylpropanolamine
       *pseudoephedrine

methyldopa
Aldoclor, Aldomet, Aldoril

Severity: ●●○
Probability: ●○○

USES: Sympathomimetics are used to treat shock; those marked with an asterisk are used in nonprescription cold and appetite suppressant products (read labels). Methyldopa is used for high blood pressure.

EFFECT: The effect of sympathomimetics may be increased.

RESULT: Increased risk of adverse effects such as heart beat irregularities, dangerous rise in blood pressure, headache, fever, visual disturbances.

WHAT TO DO: Monitor blood pressure and symptoms. Discontinue the sympathomimetic if necessary.

240. **sympathomimetics**
     ↑ Direct-acting
       dobutamine
       epinephrine
       methoxamine
       Norepinephrine
       *phenylephrine
     ↓ Mixed or indirect-acting
       dopamine
       *ephedrine
       mephentermine
       metaraminol
       *phenylpropanolamine
       *pseudoephedrine

reserpine
Demi-Regroton
Diupres
Diutensen-R
Hydromox R
Hydropres
Regroton
Renese-R
Salutensin
Ser-Ap-Es
Serpasil

Severity: ●●○
Probability: ●○○

USES: Sympathomimetics are used to treat shock; those marked with an asterisk are used in nonprescription cold and appetite suppressant products (read labels). Reserpine is used for high blood pressure.

EFFECT: The effect of direct-acting sympathomimetics may be increased. The effect of mixed or indirect-acting sympathomimetics may be decreased.

RESULT: Direct-acting sympathomimetics: increased risk of adverse effects such as heart beat irregularities, dangerous rise in blood pressure, headache, fever, visual disturbances. Mixed or indirect-acting sympathomimetics: the condition treated may not be properly controlled.

WHAT TO DO: Monitor blood pressure, symptoms, and patient response. Depending on the sympathomimetic used, the dose may need to be decreased or increased.

241. ↓ **sympathomimetics**   **urinary acidifiers**
    ephedrine   ammonium chloride
    pseudoephedrine   Ipsatol Expectorant Syrup
                                           P-V-Tussin Syrup
                                         Quelidrine Syrup
                                potassium acid phosphate
                                         K-Phos
                                       K-Phos No. 2
                                       Thiacide
                                  sodium acid phosphate
                                       K-Phos No. 2
                                     Uroqid-Acid
                                     Uroqid-Acid No. 2

Severity: ●○○
Probability: ●○○

USES: Ephedrine and pseudoephedrine are used as nasal decongestants in some nonprescription cold/cough products. Urinary acidifiers: ammonium chloride is an expectorant (agent which liquefies mucus) and is used in some cough syrups; potassium acid phosphate and sodium acid phosphate are used to make the urine more acidic.

EFFECT: The effect of the sympathomimetic may be decreased.

RESULT: The condition treated with the sympathomimetic may not be properly controlled.

WHAT TO DO: Monitor the clinical response and use a higher dose of the sympathomimetic as needed.

242. ↑ **sympathomimetics**
  ephedrine
  pseudoephedrine

urinary alkalinizers
potassium citrate
  Alka-Seltzer
  K-Lyte
sodium acetate
sodium bicarbonate
  Alka-Seltzer
  Citrocarbonate
sodium citrate
  Alka-Seltzer
sodium lactate
tromethamine

  Severity: ●●○
Probability: ●○○

USES: Ephedrine and pseudoephedrine are used as nasal decongestants in some nonprescription cold/cough products. Urinary alkalinizers are used in some antacids and in some potassium supplement products.

EFFECT: The effect of the sympathomimetic may be increased.

RESULT: Increased risk of adverse effects such as heart beat irregularities, dangerous rise in blood pressure, headache, fever, visual disturbances.

WHAT TO DO: Watch for symptoms and lower the dose of the sympathomimetic as needed.

243. ↓ **tetracyclines**
  demeclocycline (Declomycin)
  doxycycline
    Doryx, Vibramycin
    Vibra-tab
  methacycline
    Rondomycin
  minocycline (Minocin)

aluminum
aluminum carbonate
aluminum hydroxide
aluminum phosphate
attapulgite
dihydroxyaluminum
  aminoacetate
dihydroxyaluminum sodium

oxytetracycline (Terramycin)   carbonate
tetracycline   kaolin
   Achromycin V, Sumycin   magaldrate
    Brand names:
     AlternaGEL, Aludrox
     Amphojel, Basaljel
     Camalox, Creamalin
     Delcid, Di-Gel, Gaviscon
     Gelusil, Kaopectate
     Kudrox, Maalox, Mylanta
     Phosphaljel, Riopan
     Rolaids, Tempo, WinGel

Severity: ●●○
Probability: ●●○

USES: Tetracycline is an antibiotic used for microbial infections. Aluminum salts are used in various over-the-counter antacids (read product labels) and in Kaopectate (for diarrhea).

EFFECT: The effect of tetracycline may be decreased.

RESULT: The condition treated with tetracycline may not be properly controlled.

WHAT TO DO: Take the two drugs 3-4 hours apart.

244. ↓ **tetracyclines**   **bismuth**
   demeclocycline (Declomycin)   bismuth hydroxide
   doxycycline   bismuth subcarbonate
    Doryx, Vibramycin   bismuth subgallate (Devrom)
    Vibra-tab   bismuth subsalicylate
   methacycline (Rondomycin)   Pepto-Bismol
   minocycline (Minocin)
   oxytetracycline (Terramycin)
   tetracycline
    Achromycin V, Sumycin

Severity: ●●○
Probability: ●○○

USES: Tetracycline is an antibiotic used for microbial infections. Bismuth salts are used in nonprescription products for diarrhea.

EFFECT: The effect of tetracycline may be decreased.

RESULT: The condition treated with tetracycline may not be properly controlled.

WHAT TO DO: Take the two drugs 3-4 hours apart.

245. ↓ **tetracyclines**   **calcium**

demeclocycline (Declomycin)   calcium carbonate
doxycycline   calcium citrate
  Doryx, Vibramycin   calcium glubionate
  Vibra-tab   calcium gluconate
methacycline (Rondomycin)   calcium lactate
minocycline (Minocin)   calcium phosphate
oxytetracycline (Terramycin)   tricalcium phosphate
tetracycline   *Brand names*:
  Achromycin V, Sumycin   Cal-Bid, Cal-Plus, Calcet
    Calel-D, Caltrate, Citracal
    Dical, Fosfree, Iromin-G
    Mission Prenatal, Natalins
    Neo-Calglucon, Os-Cal
    Posture, Pramet FA
    Pramilet FA, Zenate

Severity: ●●○
Probability: ●●○

USES: Tetracycline is an antibiotic used for microbial infections. Calcium products are used as calcium supplements.

EFFECT: The effect of tetracycline may be decreased. (Note: doxycycline interacts minimally.)

RESULT: The condition treated with tetracycline may not be properly controlled.

WHAT TO DO: Take the two drugs 3-4 hours apart.

246. ↓ **tetracyclines**   **food**

demeclocycline (Declomycin)   food and milk
doxycycline
  Doryx, Vibramycin
  Vibra-tab
methacycline (Rondomycin)
minocycline (Minocin)
oxytetracycline (Terramycin)
tetracycline
  Achromycin V, Sumycin

Severity: ●●○
Probability: ●●○

USES: Tetracycline is an antibiotic used for microbial infections.

EFFECT: The effect of tetracycline may be decreased. (Note: doxycycline and minocycline interact minimally.)

RESULT: The condition treated with tetracycline may not be properly controlled.

WHAT TO DO: Take tetracycline at least one hour before or two hours after meals or milk. (Note: It may be best to take doxycycline, which interacts minimally, with food to reduce the likelihood of stomach irritation.)

247. ↓ **tetracyclines**
demeclocycline (Declomycin)
doxycycline
   Doryx, Vibramycin
   Vibra-tab
methacycline (Rondomycin)
minocycline (Minocin)
oxytetracycline (Terramycin)
tetracycline
   Achromycin V, Sumycin

Iron
ferrous fumarate
ferrous gluconate
ferrous sulfate
iron polysaccharide
Brand names:
   Caltrate, Chromagen, Feosol
   Feostat, Ferancee, Fergon
   Fero-Folic-500, Fero-Grad-500
   Ferralet, Ferro-Sequels
   Fosfree, Hemocyte, Hytinic
   Iberet, Ircon, Iromin-G
   Mission Prenatal, Mol-Iron
   Natalins Rx, Poly-Vi-Flor
   Pramet FA, Pramilet FA
   Simron, Slow Fe, Stuartinic
   Trinsicon, Zenate

Severity: ●●○
Probability: ●●○

USES: Tetracycline is an antibiotic used for microbial infections. Iron products are used as iron supplements.

EFFECT: The effect of tetracycline may be decreased.

RESULT: The condition treated with tetracycline may not be properly controlled.

WHAT TO DO: Take the two drugs 3-4 hours apart. (Note: Enteric-coated and sustained-release iron preparations interact to a lesser extent than other iron formulations.)

248. ↓ **tetracyclines**   **magnesium**

demeclocycline (Declomycin)   magaldrate
doxycycline   magnesium carbonate
  Doryx, Vibramycin   magnesium citrate
  Vibra-tab   magnesium gluconate
methacycline (Rondomycin)   magnesium hydroxide
minocycline (Minocin)   magnesium oxide
oxytetracycline (Terramycin)   magnesium sulfate
tetracycline   magnesium trisilicate
  Achromycin V, Sumycin   *Brand names*:
                                   Alkets, Aludrox, BiSoDol
                                   Camalox, Citroma
                                   Delcid, Di-Gel, Epsom salts
                                   Gaviscon, Gelusil
                                   Haley's M-O, Kudrox
                                   Maalox, Mag-Ox, Magonate
                                   Marblen, milk of magnesia
                                   Mylanta, Riopan, Silain-Gel
                                   Tempo, Uro-Mag, WinGel

Severity: ●●○
Probability: ●●○

USES: Tetracycline is an antibiotic used for microbial infections. Magnesium salts are used in nonprescription antacid and laxative products.

EFFECT: The effect of tetracycline may be decreased.

RESULT: The condition treated with tetracycline may not be properly controlled.

WHAT TO DO: Take the two drugs 3-4 hours apart.

249. ↓ **tetracyclines**   **urinary alkalinizers**

demeclocycline (Declomycin)   potassium citrate
doxycycline   Alka-Seltzer
  Doryx, Vibramycin   K-Lyte
  Vibra-tab   sodium acetate
methacycline (Rondomycin)   sodium bicarbonate
minocycline (Minocin)   Alka-Seltzer
oxytetracycline (Terramycin)   Citrocarbonate
tetracycline   sodium citrate
  Achromycin V, Sumycin   Alka-Seltzer
                                 sodium lactate
                                 tromethamine

Severity: ●●○
Probability: ●○○

USES: Tetracycline is an antibiotic used for microbial infections. Urinary alkalinizers are used in some antacids and in some potassium supplement products.

EFFECT: The effect of tetracycline may be decreased.

RESULT: The condition treated with tetracycline may not be properly controlled.

WHAT TO DO: Use a higher dose of tetracycline as necessary. Taking the two drugs 3-4 hours apart may help minimize this interaction.

250. ↓ **tetracyclines**   **zinc**
demeclocycline (Declomycin)   zinc gluconate
doxycycline   zinc sulfate
  Doryx, Vibramycin   Eldercaps, Eldertonic
  Vibra-tab   Glutofac, Hemocyte Plus
methacycline (Rondomycin)   Orazinc, Vi-Zac, Vicon
minocycline (Minocin)
oxytetracycline (Terramycin)
tetracycline
  Achromycin V, Sumycin

Severity: ●●○
Probability: ●●○

USES: Tetracycline is an antibiotic used for microbial infections. Zinc products are used as zinc supplements.

EFFECT: The effect of tetracycline may be decreased.

RESULT: The condition treated with tetracycline may not be properly controlled.

WHAT TO DO: Take the two drugs 3-4 hours apart. Option: take doxycycline, which may not interact or may interact only minimally.

251. ↑ **theophyllines**   **antibiotics, quinolone**
aminophylline   ciprofloxacin (Cipro)
  Somophyllin   enoxacin (Comprecin)
dyphylline   norfloxacin (Noroxin)
  Dilor, Lufyllin   ofloxacin (Floxin)
oxtriphylline
  Choledyl

theophylline
Aerolate, Bronkodyl
Bronkaid, Constant-T
Elixophyllin, Marax, Mudrane
Primatene, Quibron, Respbid
Slo-bid, Slo-Phyllin, T-PHYL
Tedral, Theo-24, Theo-Dur
Theo-Organidin, Theobid
Theolair, Theospan-SR
Theostat 80, Uniphyl

Severity: ●●○
Probability: ●●○

USES: Theophyllines are used for asthma and for bronchospasm associated with chronic bronchitis and emphysema. Quinolone antibiotics are used for microbial infections.

EFFECT: The effect of theophylline may be increased.

RESULT: Increased risk of theophylline toxicity with symptoms such as tremors, rapid heart beat, heart beat irregularities, nausea, dizziness, headache, irritability, possible seizures.

WHAT TO DO: Monitor theophylline blood levels and symptoms, and lower the dose of theophylline as needed.

252. ↓ **theophyllines**
aminophylline
Somophyllin
oxtriphylline
Choledyl
theophylline
Aerolate, Bronkodyl
Bronkaid, Constant-T
Elixophyllin, Marax, Mudrane
Primatene, Quibron, Respbid
Slo-bid, Slo-Phyllin, T-PHYL
Tedral, Theo-24, Theo-Dur
Theo-Organidin, Theobid
Theolair, Theospan-SR
Theostat 80, Uniphyl

barbiturates
amobarbital (Amytal)
aprobarbital (Alurate)
butabarbital (Butisol)
butalbital
mephobarbital (Mebaral)
pentobarbital (Nembutal)
phenobarbital
primidone (Mysoline)
secobarbital (Seconal)
talbutal (Lotusate)

Severity: ●●○
Probability: ●○○

USES: Theophyllines are used for asthma and for bronchospasm associated with chronic bronchitis and emphysema. Barbiturates are used as sedatives or sleep inducers; phenobarbital and primidone are used for seizure disorders such as epilepsy.

EFFECT: The effect of theophylline may be decreased.

RESULT: The condition treated with theophylline may not be properly controlled.

WHAT TO DO: Monitor theophylline blood levels and clinical response, and use a higher dose of theophylline as needed. Option: dyphylline (Dilor, Lufyllin) may not interact.

253. ↓ **theophyllines**

aminophylline
  Somophyllin
dyphylline
  Dilor, Lufyllin
oxtriphylline
  Choledyl
theophylline
  Aerolate, Bronkodyl
  Bronkaid, Constant-T
  Elixophyllin, Marax, Mudrane
  Primatene, Quibron, Respbid
  Slo-bid, Slo-Phyllin, T-PHYL
  Tedral, Theo-24, Theo-Dur
  Theo-Organidin, Theobid
  Theolair, Theospan-SR
  Theostat 80, Uniphyl

beta blockers (non-selective)

carteolol (Cartrol)
nadolol (Corgard)
penbutolol (Levatol)
pindolol (Visken)
propranolol (Inderal)
timolol (Blocadren)

Severity: ●●○
Probability: ●●○

USES: Theophyllines are used for asthma and for bronchospasm associated with chronic bronchitis and emphysema. Beta blockers are used for high blood pressure, angina heart pain, and irregular heart beats. Some have other uses, such as in the prevention of migraine headache and to calm the physical manifestations of "stage fright."

EFFECT: The therapeutic effect of theophylline may be antagonized.

RESULT: The condition treated with theophylline may not be properly controlled.

WHAT TO DO: Monitor theophylline blood levels and clinical response, and adjust the theophylline dose as needed. Option: use a cardioselective beta blocker such as acebutolol (Sectral), atenolol (Tenormin), betaxolol (Kerlone), esmolol (Brevibloc), or metoprolol (Lopressor). (Note: In high doses, cardioselectivity is lost.)

254. **↑ theophyllines**
aminophylline
  Somophyllin
oxtriphylline
  Choledyl
theophylline
  Aerolate, Bronkodyl
  Bronkaid, Constant-T
  Elixophyllin, Marax, Mudrane
  Primatene, Quibron, Respbid
  Slo-bid, Slo-Phyllin, T-PHYL
  Tedral, Theo-24, Theo-Dur
  Theo-Organidin, Theobid
  Theolair, Theospan-SR
  Theostat 80, Uniphyl

birth control pills
Brevicon, Demulen, Genora
Levlen, Lo-Ovral, Loestrin
Modicon, Nelova, Norcept
Nordette, Norethin, Norinyl
Norlestrin, Ortho-Novum
Ovcon, Ovral
Tri-Levlen, Tri-Norinyl

Severity: ●●○
Probability: ●○○

USES: Theophyllines are used for asthma and for bronchospasm associated with chronic bronchitis and emphysema. Birth control pills are used to prevent pregnancy.

EFFECT: The effect of theophylline may be increased.

RESULT: Increased risk of theophylline toxicity with symptoms such as tremors, rapid heart beat, heart beat irregularities, nausea, dizziness, headache, irritability, possible seizures.

WHAT TO DO: Monitor theophylline blood levels and symptoms, and lower the dose of theophylline as needed.

255. **↑ theophyllines**
aminophylline
  Somophyllin
oxtriphylline
  Choledyl

cimetidine (Tagamet)

theophylline
  Aerolate, Bronkodyl
  Bronkaid, Constant-T
  Elixophyllin, Marax, Mudrane
  Primatene, Quibron, Respbid
  Slo-bid, Slo-Phyllin, T-PHYL
  Tedral, Theo-24, Theo-Dur
  Theo-Organidin, Theobid
  Theolair, Theospan-SR
  Theostat 80, Uniphyl

Severity: ●●○
Probability: ●●●

USES: Theophyllines are used for asthma and for bronchospasm associated with chronic bronchitis and emphysema. Cimetidine is used for duodenal and gastric ulcers.

EFFECT: The effect of theophylline may be increased.

RESULT: Increased risk of theophylline toxicity with symptoms such as tremors, rapid heart beat, heart beat irregularities, nausea, dizziness, headache, irritability, possible seizures.

WHAT TO DO: Monitor theophylline blood levels and symptoms, and lower the dose (by 20-40% usually) of theophylline as needed.

256. ↑ **theophyllines**   **disulfiram (Antabuse)**
aminophylline
  Somophyllin
oxtriphylline
  Choledyl
theophylline
  Aerolate, Bronkodyl
  Bronkaid, Constant-T
  Elixophyllin, Marax, Mudrane
  Primatene, Quibron, Respbid
  Slo-bid, Slo-Phyllin, T-PHYL
  Tedral, Theo-24, Theo-Dur,
  Theo-Organidin, Theobid
  Theolair, Theospan-SR
  Theostat 80, Uniphyl

Severity: ●●○
Probability: ●○○

USES: Theophyllines are used for asthma and for bronchospasm associated with chronic bronchitis and emphysema. Disulfiram is prescribed to deter ingestion of alcoholic beverages.

EFFECT: The effect of theophylline may be increased.

RESULT: Increased risk of theophylline toxicity with symptoms such as tremors, rapid heart beat, heart beat irregularities, nausea, dizziness, headache, irritability, possible seizures.

WHAT TO DO: Monitor theophylline blood levels and symptoms, and lower the dose of theophylline as needed.

257. ↑ **theophyllines**
aminophylline
  Somophyllin
oxtriphylline
  Choledyl
theophylline
  Aerolate, Bronkodyl
  Bronkaid, Constant-T
  Elixophyllin, Marax, Mudrane
  Primatene, Quibron, Respbid
  Slo-bid, Slo-Phyllin, T-PHYL
  Tedral, Theo-24, Theo-Dur
  Theo-Organidin, Theobid
  Theolair, Theospan-SR
  Theostat 80, Uniphyl

↓ **erythromycin**
E.E.S., E-Mycin, Ery-Tab
Eryc, EryPed, Erythrocin
Eryzole, Ilosone, Ilotycin
Pediazole
troleandomycin (Tao)

Severity: ●●○
Probability: ●●●

USES: Theophyllines are used for asthma and for bronchospasm associated with chronic bronchitis and emphysema. Erythromycin and troleandomycin are antibiotics used for microbial infections.

EFFECT: The effect of theophylline may be increased. The effect of erythromycin and troleandomycin may be decreased.

RESULT: Theophylline: increased risk of theophylline toxicity with symptoms such as tremors, rapid heart beat, heart beat irregularities, nausea, dizziness, headache, irritability, possible seizures. Erythromycin and troleandomycin: the condition treated may not be properly controlled.

WHAT TO DO: Monitor theophylline blood levels and symptoms, and lower the dose of theophylline as needed. Increase the dose of erythromycin or troleandomycin if necessary.

258.   theophyllines   food
    Aerolate, Bronkodyl
    Bronkaid, Constant-T
    Elixophyllin, Marax, Mudrane
    Primatene, Quibron, Respbid
    Slo-bid, Slo-Phyllin, T-PHYL
    Tedral, Theo-24, Theo-Dur
    Theo-Organidin, Theobid
    Theolair, Theospan-SR
    Theostat 80, Uniphyl

Severity: ●●○
Probability: ●○○

USES: Theophyllines are used for asthma and for bronchospasm associated with chronic bronchitis and emphysema.

EFFECT: This interaction is complex and depends on the type of diet. The effect of theophylline may be decreased by a high protein diet and increased by a low-protein diet. Also, large amounts of charcoal-broiled beef may decrease the effect of theophylline. Food may not significantly alter the effect of an immediate-release theophylline formulation and may or may not alter the effect of a timed-release formulation, depending on the particular product. Food has little effect on Theo-Dur tablets, Theobid capsules, and Slo-bid Gyrocaps.

RESULT: Increased theophylline effect: increased risk of theophylline toxicity with symptoms such as tremors, rapid heart beat, heart beat irregularities, nausea, dizziness, headache, irritabilty, possible seizures. Decreased theophylline effect: the condition treated with theophylline may not be properly controlled.

WHAT TO DO: Monitor theophylline blood levels and alter the dosage schedule as warranted.

259. ↓ theophyllines   ↓ phenytoin (Dilantin)
    aminophylline   ethotoin (Peganone)
      Somophyllin   mephenytoin (Mesantoin)
    oxtriphylline
      Choledyl
    theophylline
      Aerolate, Bronkodyl
      Bronkaid, Constant-T
      Elixophyllin, Marax, Mudrane
      Primatene, Quibron, Respbid

Slo-bid, Slo-Phyllin, T-PHYL
Tedral, Theo-24, Theo-Dur
Theo-Organidin, Theobid
Theolair, Theospan-SR
Theostat 80, Uniphyl

Severity: ●●○
Probability: ●●○

USES: Theophyllines are used for asthma and for bronchospasm associated with chronic bronchitis and emphysema. Phenytoin is an anticonvulsant drug used for seizure disorders such as epilepsy.

EFFECT: The effect of both theophylline and phenytoin may be decreased.

RESULT: The conditions treated with the drugs may not be properly controlled.

WHAT TO DO: Monitor theophylline and phenytoin blood levels and clinical response, and adjust doses of both drugs as needed.

260. ↓ **theophyllines**   **rifampin**
aminophylline   Rifadin
Somophyllin   Rifamate
oxtriphylline   Rimactane
Choledyl   Rimactane/INH
theophylline
Aerolate, Bronkodyl
Bronkaid, Constant-T
Elixophyllin, Marax, Mudrane
Primatene, Quibron, Respbid
Slo-bid, Slo-Phyllin, T-PHYL
Tedral, Theo-24, Theo-Dur
Theo-Organidin, Theobid
Theolair, Theospan-SR
Theostat 80, Uniphyl

Severity: ●●○
Probability: ●●○

USES: Theophyllines are used for asthma and for bronchospasm associated with chronic bronchitis and emphysema. Rifampin is a specialized antibiotic used for tuberculosis and may also be given to suspected meningitis carriers.

EFFECT: The effect of theophylline may be decreased.

RESULT: The condition treated with theophylline may not be properly controlled.

WHAT TO DO: Monitor theophylline blood levels and clinical response, and use a higher dose of theophylline as needed.

261. theophyllines   **thioamines**
aminophylline   methimazole (Tapazole)
  Somophyllin   propylthiouracil (PTU)
oxtriphylline
  Choledyl
theophylline
  Aerolate, Bronkodyl
  Bronkaid, Constant-T
  Elixophyllin, Marax, Mudrane
  Primatene, Quibron, Respbid
  Slo-bid, Slo-Phyllin, T-PHYL
  Tedral, Theo-24, Theo-Dur
  Theo-Organidin, Theobid
  Theolair, Theospan-SR
  Theostat 80, Uniphyl

Severity: ●●○
Probability: ●○○

USES: Theophyllines are used for asthma and for bronchospasm associated with chronic bronchitis and emphysema. Thioamines are antithyroid agents used for hyperthyroidism.

EFFECT: The effect of theophylline may be increased in hypothyroid patients and decreased in hyperthyroid patients. Once a patient is made euthyroid (normal thyroid gland function), the theophylline effect is normal.

RESULT: Increased theophylline effect: increased risk of theophylline toxicity with symptoms such as tremors, rapid heart beat, heart beat irregularities, nausea, dizziness, headache, irritability, possible seizures. Decreased theophylline effect: the condition treated may not be properly controlled.

WHAT TO DO: Monitor theophylline blood levels and symptoms, and adjust the dose of theophylline as needed. Maintaining the patient in the euthyroid state is necessary for normal theophylline effect.

262. **theophyllines**
aminophylline
  Somophyllin
oxtriphylline
  Choledyl
theophylline
  Aerolate, Bronkodyl
  Bronkaid, Constant-T
  Elixophyllin, Marax, Mudrane
  Primatene, Quibron, Respbid
  Slo-bid, Slo-Phyllin, T-PHYL
  Tedral, Theo-24, Theo-Dur
  Theo-Organidin, Theobid
  Theolair, Theospan-SR
  Theostat 80, Uniphyl

thyroid
dextrothyroxine (Choloxin)
levothyroxine (Synthroid)
liothyronine (Cytomel)
liotrix (Euthroid, Thyrolar)
thyroglobulin (Proloid)
thyroid (Armour Thyroid)

Severity: ●●○
Probability: ●○○

USES: Theophyllines are used for asthma and for bronchospasm associated with chronic bronchitis and emphysema. Thyroid hormones are used for hypothyroidism and for goiters (enlargements of the thyroid gland).

EFFECT: The effect of theophylline may be increased in hypothyroid patients and decreased in hyperthyroid patients. Once a patient is made euthyroid (normal thyroid gland function), the theophylline effect is normal.

RESULT: Increased theophylline effect: increased risk of theophylline toxicity with symptoms such as tremors, rapid heart beat, heart beat irregularities, nausea, dizziness, headache, irritability, possible seizures. Decreased theophylline effect: the condition treated may not be properly controlled.

WHAT TO DO: Monitor theophylline blood levels and symptoms, and adjust the dose of theophylline as needed. Maintaining the patient in the euthyroid state is necessary for normal theophylline effect.

263. ↑ **theophyllines**
aminophylline
  Somophyllin
oxtriphylline
  Choledyl

ticlopidine (Ticlid)

theophylline
  Aerolate, Bronkodyl
  Bronkaid, Constant-T
  Elixophyllin, Marax, Mudrane
  Primatene, Quibron, Respbid
  Slo-bid, Slo-Phyllin, T-PHYL
  Tedral, Theo-24, Theo-Dur
  Theo-Organidin, Theobid
  Theolair, Theospan-SR
  Theostat 80, Uniphyl

Severity: ●●○
Probability: ●○○

USES: Theophyllines are used for asthma and for bronchospasm associated with chronic bronchitis and emphysema. Ticlopidine is a "blood thinner" used to reduce the risk of stroke in high-risk patients and for other conditions.

EFFECT: The effect of theophylline may be increased.

RESULT: Increased risk of theophylline toxicity with symptoms such as tremors, rapid heart beat, heart beat irregularities, nausea, dizziness, headache, irritability, possible seizures.

WHAT TO DO: Monitor theophylline blood levels and symptoms, and lower the dose of theophylline as needed.

264. ↑ **theophyllines**   **verapamil**
                                             (Calan, Isoptin)

aminophylline
  Somophyllin
oxtriphylline
  Choledyl
theophylline
  Aerolate, Bronkodyl
  Bronkaid, Constant-T
  Elixophyllin, Marax, Mudrane
  Primatene, Quibron, Respbid
  Slo-bid, Slo-Phyllin, T-PHYL
  Tedral, Theo-24, Theo-Dur
  Theo-Organidin, Theobid
  Theolair, Theospan-SR
  Theostat 80, Uniphyl

Severity: ●●○
Probability: ●○○

USES: Theophyllines are used for asthma and for bronchospasm associated with chronic bronchitis and emphysema. Verapamil is a calcium channel blocker used for high blood pressure, angina heart pain, and heart beat irregularities.

EFFECT: The effect of theophylline may be increased.

RESULT: Increased risk of theophylline toxicity with symptoms such as tremors, rapid heart beat, heart beat irregularities, nausea, dizziness, headache, irritability, possible seizures.

WHAT TO DO: Monitor theophylline blood levels and symptoms, and lower the dose of theophylline as needed.

---

265. ↑ **thiopurines, oral**   **allopurinol (Zyloprim)**
azathioprine (Imuran)
mercaptopurine (Purinethol)

Severity: ●●●
Probability: ●●●

USES: Azathioprine is used for prevention of rejection in kidney transplantation and for severe rheumatoid arthritis. Mercaptopurine is used for acute lymphatic leukemia. Allopurinol is used for gout and in certain types of cancer therapy.

EFFECT: The effect of the thiopurine may be increased.

RESULT: Increased risk of adverse effects such as blood disorders and nausea and vomiting.

WHAT TO DO: Lower the starting thiopurine dose (by 65-75%) and adjust as needed thereafter based on clinical response and adverse symptoms.

---

266. ↓ **thyroid**   **cholestyramine
(Questran)**

dextrothyroxine (Choloxin)
levothyroxine (Synthroid)
liothyronine (Cytomel)
liotrix (Euthroid, Thyrolar)
thyroglobulin (Proloid)
thyroid (Armour Thyroid)

Severity: ●●○
Probability: ●○○

USES: Thyroid hormones are used for hypothyroidism and for goiters (enlargements of the thyroid gland). Cholestyramine is used to lower cholesterol blood levels.

EFFECT: The effect of thyroid may be decreased.

RESULT: The condition treated with thyroid may not be properly controlled.

WHAT TO DO: Take the two drugs at least six hours apart.

267. ↓ **tocainide (Tonocard)**　　　　**rifampin**
Rifadin
Rifamate
Rimactane
Rimactane/INH

Severity: ●●○
Probability: ●○○

USES: Tocainide is used for life-threatening heart beat irregularities of the ventricular type. Rifampin is a specialized antibiotic used for tuberculosis and may also be given to suspected meningitis carriers.

EFFECT: The effect of tocainide may be decreased.

RESULT: The condition treated with tocainide may not be properly controlled.

WHAT TO DO: Monitor tocainide blood levels and clinical response, and adjust the dose of tocainide as needed.

268. ↓ **valproic acid**　　　　　　↑ **carbamazepine**
　　　 (Depakene)　　　　　　　 **(Epitol, tegretol)**

Severity: ●●○
Probability: ●○○

USES: Valproic acid is an anticonvulsant drug used for seizure disorders such as epilepsy. Carbamazepine is an anticonvulsant drug used for seizure disorders such as epilepsy, and is also used for certain types of neuralgia (nerve pain).

EFFECT: The effect of valproic acid may be decreased. The effect of carbamazepine may be increased, but this effect may be inconsistent.

RESULT: Valproic acid: the condition treated may not be properly controlled. Carbamazepine: possible increased risk of adverse effects such as dizziness, drowsiness, unsteadiness, nausea and vomiting.

WHAT TO DO: Monitor blood levels of both drugs, clinical response, and symptoms, and adjust the dose of both drugs as needed.

269. ↑ valproic acid **salicylates**
      (Depakene)

                                              aspirin
    Alka Seltzer, Anacin
    Ascriptin, Aspergum, Bayer
    Bufferin, Cama, Ecotrin
    Empirin, Measurin,
    Momentum, Persistin
    St. Joseph
bismuth subsalicylate
    Pepto Bismol
choline salicylate
    Arthropan
magnesium salicylate
    Doan's
salsalate (Disalcid)
sodium salicylate (Uracel)
sodium thiosalicylate
    Tusal

Severity: ●●○
Probability: ●○○

USES: Valproic acid is an anticonvulsant drug used for seizure disorders such as epilepsy. Salicylates are used for arthritic-type conditions and for general pain, fever, and inflammation.

EFFECT: The effect of valproic acid may be increased.

RESULT: Increased risk of adverse effects such as nausea, vomiting, indigestion, headache, visual disturbances, tremors, loss of muscle coordination.

WHAT TO DO: Monitor valproic acid blood levels and liver enzymes, and watch for symptoms. Lower the dose of valproic acid as needed.

270. ↓ **verapamil**   **calcium**
         (Calan, Isoptin)

calcium carbonate
calcium citrate
calcium glubionate
calcium gluconate
calcium lactate
calcium phosphate
tricalcium phosphate
Brand names:
  Cal-Bid, Cal-Plus, Calcet
  Calel-D, Caltrate, Citracal
  Dical, Fosfree, Iromin-G
  Mission Prenatal, Natalins
  Neo-Calglucon, Os-Cal
  Posture, Pramet FA
  Pramilet FA, Zenate

Severity: ●●○
Probability: ●○○

USES: Verapamil is a calcium channel blocker used for high blood pressure, angina heart pain, and heart beat irregularities. Calcium salts are used in nonprescription calcium supplements and in some antacids (read product labels).

EFFECT: The effect of verapamil may be antagonized by calcium.

RESULT: The condition treated with verapamil may not be properly controlled.

WHAT TO DO: Monitor the patient for loss of verapamil effectiveness.

271.   **verapamil**   ↑ **quinidine**
           (Calan, Isoptin)

Cardioquin, Cin-Quin
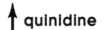
Duraquin
Quinaglute Dura-Tabs
Quinalan, Quinidex Extentabs
Quinora

Severity: ●●●
Probability: ●○○

USES: Verapamil is a calcium channel blocker used for high blood pressure, angina heart pain, and heart beat irregularities. Quinidine is used for heart beat irregularities.

EFFECT: The effect of quinidine may be increased with toxic effects.

RESULT: Increased risk of adverse effects such as a fall in blood pressure, slowed heart beat, heart beat irregularities, and fluid in the lungs.

WHAT TO DO: Monitor quinidine blood levels and symptoms, and stop this combination if warranted. Avoid this combination unless no alternatives are feasible.

272. ↓ **verapamil**   **rifampin**
         (Calan, Isoptin)
                                          Rifadin
                                          Rifamate
                                          Rimactane
                                          Rimactane/INH

     Severity: ●●○
Probability: ●○○

USES: Verapamil is a calcium channel blocker used for high blood pressure, angina heart pain, and heart beat irregularities. Rifampin is a specialized antibiotic used for tuberculosis and may also be given to suspected meningitis carriers.

EFFECT: The effect of orally-administered verapamil may be decreased.

RESULT: The condition treated with verapamil may not be properly controlled.

WHAT TO DO: If feasible, use an alternative to either verapamil or rifampin. Option: use intravenous verapamil, which does not interact.

273. ↓ **vitamin A**   **aminoglycosides**
                                          kanamycin (Kantrex)
                                          neomycin
                                            Mycifradin, Neobiotic
                                          paromomycin (Humatin)

     Severity: ●○○
Probability: ●○○

USES: Vitamin A is essential for healthy skin, hair, epithelial structures, and for adequate vision in dim light. Sources: milk, cream, butter, fortified margarine, egg yolk, green leafy and yellow vegetables, and fish liver oils; also available in numerous vitamin supplements (read product labels). Aminoglycosides are a specialized type of antibiotic.

EFFECT: The effect of vitamin A may be decreased.

RESULT: Vitamin A ingested through diet or supplementation may not be absorbed by the body as well as expected.

WHAT TO DO: Take a vitamin A supplement and an aminoglycoside several hours apart.

274. ↓ **vitamin A**   **mineral oil**
                                        Fleet Mineral Oil Enema
                                        Haley's M-O
                                        mineral oil (various brands)

Severity: ●○○
Probability: ●○○

USES: Vitamin A is essential for healthy skin, hair, epithelial structures, and for adequate vision in dim light. Sources: milk, cream, butter, fortified margarine, egg yolk, green leafy and yellow vegetables, and fish liver oils; also available in numerous vitamin supplements (read product labels). Mineral oil is used as a laxative.

EFFECT: The effect of vitamin A may be decreased.

RESULT: Vitamin A ingested through diet or supplementation may not be absorbed by the body as well as expected.

WHAT TO DO: Take a vitamin A supplement and mineral oil several hours apart. Option: use an alternative to mineral oil.

275. ↓ **vitamin B-12**   **chloramphenicol**
         cyanocobalamin injection   Chloromycetin
         various multivitamin
             products

Severity: ●○○
Probability: ●○○

USES: Vitamin B-12 promotes hemoglobin synthesis and healthy red blood cells, acts as a coenzyme in the synthesis of DNA, is essential for the proper function of nerve cells, and assists in the prevention of certain forms of anemia. Sources: liver, kidney, lean meat, eggs, milk and milk products, salt-water fish, oysters; also available in numerous vitamin supplements (read product labels). Chloramphenicol is an antibiotic used for microbial infections.

EFFECT: The effect of vitamin B-12 in patients with pernicious anemia may be decreased.

RESULT: The condition treated with vitamin B-12 may not be properly controlled.

WHAT TO DO: Monitor the clinical response. Option: use an alternative to chloramphenicol.

276. vitamin B-6 (pyridoxine) ↓ barbiturates
phenobarbital
primidone (Mysoline)

Severity: ●○○
Probability: ●○○

USES: Vitamin B-6 aids in the metabolism of proteins and fats, and is essential for proper cell function. Sources: dried yeast, liver and other organ meats, fish, vegetables, whole-grain cereals, legumes (peas, beans, etc.); also available in numerous vitamin supplements (read product labels). Phenobarbital is used as a sedative and for seizure disorders such as epilepsy; primidone is used for seizure disorders such as epilepsy.

EFFECT: The effect of phenobarbital and primidone may be decreased.

RESULT: The condition treated with the barbiturate may not be properly controlled.

WHAT TO DO: Monitor barbiturate blood levels and clinical response, and use a higher dose of barbiturate as needed.

277. vitamin B-6 (pyridoxine) ↓ phenytoin (Dilantin)

Severity: ●●○
Probability: ●○○

USES: Vitamin B-6 aids in the metabolism of proteins and fats, and is essential for proper cell function. Sources: dried yeast, liver and other organ meats, fish, vegetables, whole-grain cereals, legumes (peas, beans, etc.); also available in numerous vitamin supplements (read product labels). Phenytoin is an anticonvulsant drug used for seizure disorders such as epilepsy.

EFFECT: The effect of phenytoin may be decreased.

RESULT: The condition treated with phenytoin may not be properly controlled.

WHAT TO DO: Monitor phenytoin blood levels and clinical response, and use a higher dose of phenytoin as needed.

278.   **vitamin C**   ↓ **alcohol (ethanol)**
        (ascorbic acid)   beer, liquor, wine

        Severity: ●○○
        Probability: ●○○

USES: Vitamin C is essential for normal teeth and gums, bones, blood vessels, formation of collagen (a protein that helps support body structures), and wound healing. Sources: citrus fruits, tomatoes, potatoes, cantaloupe, berries, cabbage, green pepper, green leafy vegetables; also available in numerous vitamin supplements (read product labels).
EFFECT: The effect of alcohol may be decreased.
RESULT: The body's elimination of alcohol may be slighly increased.
WHAT TO DO: No precautions are necessary.

279.   **vitamin C**   ↓ **phenothiazines**
        (ascorbic acid)   fluphenazine (Prolixin)

        Severity: ●●○
        Probability: ●○○

USES: Vitamin C is essential for normal teeth and gums, bones, blood vessels, formation of collagen (a protein that helps support body structures), and wound healing. Sources: citrus fruits, tomatoes, potatoes, cantaloupe, berries, cabbage, green pepper, green leafy vegetables; also available in numerous vitamin supplements (read product labels). Fluphenazine is an antipsychotic drug used for brain disorders such as schizophrenia, paranoia, and manic-depressive illness.
EFFECT: The effect of fluphenazine may be decreased.
RESULT: The condition treated with fluphenazine may not be properly controlled.
WHAT TO DO: Monitor the clinical response and adjust the dose of fluphenazine as needed.

280.   vitamin C (ascorbic acid) ↓ warfarin (Coumadin)

Severity: ●●○
Probability: ●○○

USES: Vitamin C is essential for normal teeth and gums, bones, blood vessels, formation of collagen (a protein that helps support body structures), and wound healing. Sources: citrus fruits, tomatoes, potatoes, cantaloupe, berries, cabbage, green pepper, green leafy vegetables; also available in numerous vitamin supplements (read product labels). Warfarin is an anticoagulant used to thin the blood and prevent it from clotting.

EFFECT: The effect of warfarin may be decreased.

RESULT: The condition treated with warfarin may not be properly controlled.

WHAT TO DO: No precautions appear necessary unless very large doses of vitamin C (more than 5000 milligrams or 5 grams) are taken daily.

281.   ↑ vitamin D

calcifediol (Calderol)
calcitriol (Rocaltrol)
cholecalciferol (Delta-D)
dihydrotachysterol (DHT)
ergocalciferol (Calciferol)

diuretics, thiazide

bendroflumethiazide
   Naturetin
benzthiazide (Aquatag)
chlorothiazide (Diuril)
chlorthalidone (Hygroton)
cyclothiazide (Anhydron)
hydrochlorothiazide
   Esidrix, HydroDiuril
hydroflumethiazide (Saluron)
indapamide (Lozol)
methyclothiazide (Enduron)
metolazone (Diulo,
   Zaroxolyn)
polythiazide (Renese)
quinethazone (Hydromox)
trichlormethiazide (Naqua)

Severity: ●○○
Probability: ●○○

USES: Vitamin D promotes absorption of calcium and phosphorus, and is essential for normal calcification of bones and teeth. Sources: vitamin D-fortified milk, fish liver oils (especially cod liver oil), salmon, tuna, egg yolk, butter, ultraviolet light (sunlight, sunlamp); also available in numerous vitamin supplements (read product labels). Diuretics are used to rid the body of excess fluid—this makes them effective in treating congestive heart failure, high blood pressure, cirrhosis of the liver, and kidney dysfunction.

EFFECT: The effect of vitamin D may be increased.

RESULT: Increased risk of hypercalcemia (too much calcium).

WHAT TO DO: Monitor calcium blood levels and symptoms, and discontinue one or both drugs if necessary.

282.   vitamin D   ↓ **verapamil**
                                                  (Calan, Isoptin)

calcifediol (Calderol)
calcitriol (Rocaltrol)
cholecalciferol (Delta-D)
dihydrotachysterol (DHT)
ergocalciferol (Calciferol)

Severity: ●●○
Probability: ●○○

USES: Vitamin D promotes absorption of calcium and phosphorus, and is essential for normal calcification of bones and teeth. Sources: vitamin D-fortified milk, fish liver oils (especially cod liver oil), salmon, tuna, egg yolk, butter, ultraviolet light (sunlight, sunlamp); also available in numerous vitamin supplements (read product labels). Verapamil is a calcium channel blocker used for high blood pressure, angina heart pain, and heart beat irregularities.

EFFECT: The effect of verapamil may be decreased.

RESULT: The condition treated with verapamil may not be properly controlled.

WHAT TO DO: Monitor the clinical response and adjust the dose of verapamil as needed.

283.   vitamin E   ↓ **Iron**
                                                  ferrous fumarate
                                                  ferrous gluconate
                                                  ferrous sulfate
                                                  iron polysaccharide

Brand names:
Caltrate, Chromagen, Feosol
Feostat, Ferancee, Fergon
Fero-Folic-500, Fero-Grad-500
Ferralet, Ferro-Sequels
Fosfree, Hemocyte, Hytinic
Iberet, Ircon, Iromin-G
Mission Prenatal, Mol-Iron
Natalins Rx, Poly-Vi-Flor
Pramet FA, Pramilet FA
Simron, Slow Fe, Stuartinic
Trinsicon, Zenate

Severity: ●●○
Probability: ●○○

USES: Vitamin E is an important anti-oxidant needed for stability of muscle, red blood cells, and membranes, and is necessary for normal reproduction. Sources: vegetable oils, whole-grain cereals, wheat germ, green leafy vegetables, lettuce, egg yolk, margarine, legumes (peas, beans, etc.); also available in numerous vitamin supplements (read product labels). The mineral iron is an essential component of hemoglobin in the blood.

EFFECT: The effect of iron may be decreased in children with iron-deficiency anemia.

RESULT: The condition treated with iron may not be properly controlled.

WHAT TO DO: Monitor the clinical response.

---

284. ↓ **vitamin K**
phytonadione (Mephyton)

mineral oil
Fleet Mineral Oil Enema
Haley's M-O

Severity: ●○○
Probability: ●○○

USES: Vitamin K is essential for the formation of prothrombin, a substance necessary for normal blood clotting. Sources: green leafy vegetables, pork liver, vegetable oils; vitamin K also is synthesized by intestinal flora. Mineral oil is used as a laxative.

EFFECT: The effect of vitamin K may be decreased.

RESULT: The condition treated with vitamin K may not be properly controlled.

WHAT TO DO: Take vitamin K and mineral oil several hours apart. Options: 1) use an alternative to mineral oil; 2) administer vitamin K by injection.

---

285. ↓ **warfarin (Coumadin)**   **aminoglutethimide (Cytadren)**

anisindione (Miradon)
dicumarol

Severity: ●●○
Probability: ●○○

USES: Warfarin is an anticoagulant used to thin the blood and prevent it from clotting. Aminoglutethimide is used for suppression of adrenal gland function in certain patients with Cushing's syndrome.

EFFECT: The effect of warfarin may be decreased.

RESULT: The condition treated with warfarin may not be properly controlled.

WHAT TO DO: Monitor prothrombin times and use a higher dose of warfarin as needed. To prevent dangerous bleeding when this combination is stopped, the warfarin dose may need to be adjusted downward.

---

286. ↑ **warfarin (Coumadin)**   **amiodarone (Cordarone)**

Severity: ●●●
Probability: ●●●

USES: Warfarin is an anticoagulant used to thin the blood and prevent it from clotting. Amiodarone is used for heart beat irregularities.

EFFECT: The effect of warfarin may be increased. (This effect may persist for weeks after this combination is stopped.)

RESULT: Increased risk of hemorrhage with symptoms such as bruising or bleeding anywhere on the body, black or tarry stools.

WHAT TO DO: Monitor prothrombin times and lower the warfarin dose (usually 30-50% less) as needed.

287. ↑ warfarin (Coumadin)

anisindione (Miradon)
dicumarol

anabolic steroids (17-alkyl)

danazol (Danocrine)
fluoxymesterone (Halotestin)
methandrostenolone
methyltestosterone
  Android, Estratest
  Mediatric, Metandren
  Testred, Virilon
oxandrolone (Anavar)
oxymetholone (Anadrol-50)
stanozolol (Winstrol)

Severity: ●●●
Probability: ●●○

USES: Warfarin is an anticoagulant used to thin the blood and prevent it from clotting. Anabolic steroids danazol and stanozolol are used for angioedema (fluid in certain body tissues); danazol is also used for endometriosis and fibrocystic breast disease. The other steroids are used as replacement therapy in conditions associated with a deficiency of normal body testosterone (male sex hormone).

EFFECT: The effect of warfarin may be increased.

RESULT: Increased risk of hemorrhage with symptoms such as bruising or bleeding anywhere on the body, black or tarry stools.

WHAT TO DO: Monitor prothrombin times and lower the warfarin dose as needed.

288. warfarin (Coumadin)

anisindione (Miradon)
↑ dicumarol

antidepressants, tricyclic

amitriptyline (Elavil, Endep)
amoxapine (Asendin)
clomipramine (Anafranil)
desipramine
  Norpramin, Pertofrane
doxepin
  Adapin, Sinequan
imipramine (Tofranil)
nortriptyline
  Aventyl, Pamelor
protriptyline (Vivactil)
trimipramine (Surmontil)

Severity: ●●○
Probability: ●○○

USES: Dicumarol is an anticoagulant used to thin the blood and prevent it from clotting. Tricyclic antidepressants are used for clinical depression.

EFFECT: The effect of dicumarol may be increased. Warfarin appears not to interact. No information is available on anisindione.

RESULT: Increased risk of hemorrhage with symptoms such as bruising or bleeding anywhere on the body, black or tarry stools.

WHAT TO DO: Monitor prothrombin times and lower the dicumarol dose as needed.

---

289. ↓ **warfarin (Coumadin)**   **barbiturates**
  dicumarol   amobarbital (Amytal)
                                               aprobarbital (Alurate)
                                               butabarbital (Butisol)
                                               butalbital
                                               mephobarbital (Mebaral)
                                               pentobarbital (Nembutal)
                                               phenobarbital
                                               primidone (Mysoline)
                                               secobarbital (Seconal)
                                               talbutal (Lotusate)

Severity: ●●●
Probability: ●●●

USES: Warfarin is an anticoagulant used to thin the blood and prevent it from clotting. Barbiturates are used as sedatives or sleep inducers; phenobarbital and primidone are used for seizure disorders such as epilepsy.

EFFECT: The effect of warfarin may be decreased.

RESULT: The condition treated with warfarin may not be properly controlled.

WHAT TO DO: Monitor prothrombin times and use a higher dose of warfarin as needed. To prevent dangerous bleeding when this combination is stopped, adjust the warfarin dose downward. Option: use a benzodiazepine (e.g., Halcion, Valium) in place of the barbiturate.

290. ↓ **warfarin (Coumadin)**   **carbamazepine**
                                          (Epitol, Tegretol)
dicumarol

Severity: ●●○
Probability: ●○○

USES: Warfarin is an anticoagulant used to thin the blood and prevent
it from clotting. Carbamazepine is an anticonvulsant drug used for
seizure disorders such as epilepsy.

EFFECT: The effect of warfarin may be decreased.

RESULT: The condition treated with warfarin may not be properly
controlled.

WHAT TO DO: Monitor prothrombin times and use a higher dose of
warfarin as needed. To prevent dangerous bleeding when this combination is stopped, the warfarin dose may need to be adjusted downward.

291. ↑ **warfarin (Coumadin)**   **cephalosporins**
         anisindione (Miradon)   cefamandole (Mandol)
         dicumarol   cefoperazone (Cefobid)
                                            cefotetan (Cefotan)
                                            moxalactam (Moxam)

Severity: ●●●
Probability: ●○○

USES: Warfarin is an anticoagulant used to thin the blood and prevent
it from clotting. Cephalosporins are antibiotics used for microbial
infections.

EFFECT: The effect of warfarin may be increased.

RESULT: Increased risk of hemorrhage with symptoms such as bruising or bleeding anywhere on the body, black or tarry stools.

WHAT TO DO: Monitor prothrombin times and lower the warfarin
dose as needed. Taking vitamin K, which increases blood clotting,
may minimize bleeding complications.

292. ↑ **warfarin (Coumadin)**   **chloral hydrate (Noctec)**
         dicumarol

Severity: ●○○
Probability: ●●○

USES: Warfarin is an anticoagulant used to thin the blood and prevent it from clotting. Chloral hydrate is used to induce sleep.

EFFECT: The effect of warfarin may be increased. This effect is usually transient.

RESULT: Increased risk of hemorrhage with symptoms such as bruising or bleeding anywhere on the body, black or tarry stools.

WHAT TO DO: Monitor prothrombin times and lower the warfarin dose as needed. Option: use a benzodiazepine hypnotic (e.g., Halcion, Restoril) in place of chloral hydrate.

---

293. ↓ **warfarin (Coumadin)**   **cholestyramine (Questran)**

  dicumarol

  Severity: ●●○
Probability: ●●○

USES: Warfarin is an anticoagulant used to thin the blood and prevent it from clotting. Cholestyramine is used to reduce cholesterol and/or triglyceride blood levels.

EFFECT: The effect of warfarin may be decreased.

RESULT: The condition treated with warfarin may not be properly controlled.

WHAT TO DO: Take the two drugs at least 3 hours apart. Monitor prothrombin times and adjust the warfarin dose as needed. To prevent dangerous bleeding when this combination is stopped, the warfarin dose may need to be adjusted downward.

---

294. ↑ **warfarin (Coumadin)**   **cimetidine (Tagamet)**

  Severity: ●●●
Probability: ●●●

USES: Warfarin is an anticoagulant used to thin the blood and prevent it from clotting. Cimetidine is used for duodenal and gastric ulcers.

EFFECT: The effect of warfarin may be increased.

RESULT: Increased risk of hemorrhage with symptoms such as bruising or bleeding anywhere on the body, black or tarry stools.

WHAT TO DO: Monitor prothrombin times and lower the warfarin dose as needed. Avoid this combination if feasible. Option: use a non-interacting alternative to cimetidine such as nizatidine (Axid).

295. ↑ **warfarin (Coumadin)**   **clofibrate (Atromid-S)**
anisindione (Miradon)
dicumarol

Severity: ●●●
Probability: ●●●

USES: Warfarin is an anticoagulant used to thin the blood and prevent
it from clotting. Clofibrate is used to reduce cholesterol and/or
triglyceride blood levels.

EFFECT: The effect of warfarin may be increased.

RESULT: Increased risk of hemorrhage with symptoms such as bruising or bleeding anywhere on the body, black or tarry stools. Deaths
have been reported.

WHAT TO DO: Monitor prothrombin times and lower the warfarin
dose as needed. Avoid this combination if feasible.

296. ↑ **warfarin (Coumadin)**   **dextrothyroxine**
                                             (Choloxin)

anisindione (Miradon)
dicumarol

Severity: ●●●
Probability: ●●○

USES: Warfarin is an anticoagulant used to thin the blood and prevent
it from clotting. Dextrothyroxine is used to reduce cholesterol blood
levels.

EFFECT: The effect of warfarin may be increased.

RESULT: Increased risk of hemorrhage with symptoms such as bruising or bleeding anywhere on the body, black or tarry stools.

WHAT TO DO: Monitor prothrombin times and lower the warfarin
dose as needed.

297. ↑ **warfarin (Coumadin)**   **disulfiram (Antabuse)**

Severity: ●●○
Probability: ●●○

USES: Warfarin is an anticoagulant used to thin the blood and prevent
it from clotting. Disulfiram is prescribed to deter ingestion of alcoholic
beverages.

EFFECT: The effect of warfarin may be increased.

RESULT: Increased risk of hemorrhage with symptoms such as bruising or bleeding anywhere on the body, black or tarry stools.

WHAT TO DO: Monitor prothrombin times and lower the warfarin dose as needed.

298. ↑ **warfarin (Coumadin)**   **erythromycin**
                                         E.E.S., E-Mycin, Ery-Tab
                                         Eryc, EryPed, Erythroci
                                         Eryzole, Ilosone, Ilotycin
                                         Pediazole

    Severity: ●●●
Probability: ●●○

USES: Warfarin is an anticoagulant used to thin the blood and prevent it from clotting. Erythromycin is an antibiotic used for microbial infections.

EFFECT: The effect of warfarin may be increased.

RESULT: Increased risk of hemorrhage with symptoms such as bruising or bleeding anywhere on the body, black or tarry stools.

WHAT TO DO: Monitor prothrombin times and lower the warfarin dose as needed.

299. ↓ **warfarin (Coumadin)**   **ethchlorvynol (Placidyl)**
       dicumarol

    Severity: ●●○
Probability: ●○○

USES: Warfarin is an anticoagulant used to thin the blood and prevent it from clotting. Ethchlorvynol is used to induce sleep.

EFFECT: The effect of warfarin may be decreased.

RESULT: The condition treated with warfarin may not be properly controlled.

WHAT TO DO: Monitor prothrombin times and use a higher dose of warfarin as needed. To prevent dangerous bleeding when this combination is stopped, the warfarin dose may need to be adjusted downward. Option: use a benzodiazepine hypnotic (e.g., Halcion, Restoril) in place of ethchlorvynol.

300. ↑ **warfarin (Coumadin)** **glucagon**

 Severity: ●●○
Probability: ●●○

USES: Warfarin is an anticoagulant used to thin the blood and prevent it from clotting. Glucagon injection is used for severe hypoglycemic (lowered blood sugar) reactions in diabetic patients, and may also be used as a diagnostic aid in X-ray examinations.

EFFECT: The effect of warfarin may be increased.

RESULT: Increased risk of hemorrhage with symptoms such as bruising or bleeding anywhere on the body, black or tarry stools.

WHAT TO DO: Monitor prothrombin times and lower the warfarin dose as needed.

301. ↓ **warfarin (Coumadin)** **glutethimide (Doriden)**
 dicumarol

 Severity: ●●○
Probability: ●●○

USES: Warfarin is an anticoagulant used to thin the blood and prevent it from clotting. Glutethimide is used as a sedative and as a sleep inducer.

EFFECT: The effect of warfarin may be decreased.

RESULT: The condition treated with warfarin may not be properly controlled.

WHAT TO DO: Monitor prothrombin times and use a higher dose of warfarin as needed. To prevent dangerous bleeding when this combination is stopped, the warfarin dose may need to be adjusted downward. Option: use a benzodiazepine hypnotic (e.g., Doral, Halcion, Restoril) in place of glutethimide.

302. ↓ **warfarin (Coumadin)** **griseofulvin**
 Fulvicin, Grifulvin V
 Grisactin, Gris-PEG

 Severity: ●●○
Probability: ●○○

USES: Warfarin is an anticoagulant used to thin the blood and prevent it from clotting. Griseofulvin is an antifungal agent used for ringworm infections of the skin, hair, and nails and also for certain types of bacterial infections.

EFFECT: The effect of warfarin may be decreased.

RESULT: The condition treated with warfarin may not be properly controlled.

WHAT TO DO: Monitor prothrombin times and use a higher dose of warfarin as needed. To prevent dangerous bleeding when this combination is stopped, the warfarin dose may need to be adjusted downward.

303. ↑ warfarin (Coumadin)   metronidazole
Flagyl, Metryl, Protostat

Severity: ●●●
Probability: ●●●

USES: Warfarin is an anticoagulant used to thin the blood and prevent it from clotting. Metronidazole is used for trichomoniasis, a type of vaginitis, and for acute amoebic dysentery.

EFFECT: The effect of warfarin may be increased.

RESULT: Increased risk of hemorrhage with symptoms such as bruising or bleeding anywhere on the body, black or tarry stools.

WHAT TO DO: Monitor prothrombin times and lower the warfarin dose as needed.

304. ↑ warfarin (Coumadin)   phenylbutazone
(Butazolidin)

anisindione (Miradon)
dicumarol

Severity: ●●●
Probability: ●●●

USES: Warfarin is an anticoagulant used to thin the blood and prevent it from clotting. Phenylbutazone is a nonsteroidal antiinflammatory drug (NSAID) used for pain and inflammation in severe arthritic-type conditions.

EFFECT: The effect of warfarin may be increased.

RESULT: Increased risk of hemorrhage with symptoms such as bruising or bleeding anywhere on the body, black or tarry stools.

WHAT TO DO: Monitor prothrombin times and lower the warfarin dose as needed. Avoid this combination if feasible.

305. ↑ **warfarin**
anisindione (Miradon)
dicumarol

quinidine
Cardioquin, Cin-Quin
Duraquin, Quinaglute
Dura-Tabs, Quinalan
Quinidex Extentabs, Quinora

Severity: ●●●
Probability: ●○○

USES: Warfarin is an anticoagulant used to thin the blood and prevent it from clotting. Quinidine is used for heart beat irregularities.

EFFECT: The effect of warfarin may be increased.

RESULT: Increased risk of hemorrhage with symptoms such as bruising or bleeding anywhere on the body, black or tarry stools.

WHAT TO DO: Monitor prothrombin times and lower the warfarin dose as needed.

306. ↑ **warfarin (Coumadin)**
anisindione (Miradon)
dicumarol

quinine
Quin-260, Quinamm, Quine
Quinite

Severity: ●●●
Probability: ●○○

USES: Warfarin is an anticoagulant used to thin the blood and prevent it from clotting. Quinine is used for night-time leg cramps and also may be prescribed for malaria.

EFFECT: The effect of warfarin may be increased.

RESULT: Increased risk of hemorrhage with symptoms such as bruising or bleeding anywhere on the body, black or tarry stools.

WHAT TO DO: Monitor prothrombin times and lower the warfarin dose as needed. Avoid this combination if feasible.

307. ↓ **warfarin (Coumadin)**
dicumarol

rifampin
Rifadin
Rifamate
Rimactane
Rimactane/INH

Severity: ●●○
Probability: ●●●

USES: Warfarin is an anticoagulant used to thin the blood and prevent it from clotting. Rifampin is a specialized antibiotic used for tuberculosis and may also be given to suspected meningitis carriers.

EFFECT: The effect of warfarin may be decreased.

RESULT: The condition treated with warfarin may not be properly controlled.

WHAT TO DO: Monitor prothrombin times and use a higher dose of warfarin as needed. To prevent dangerous bleeding when this combination is stopped, the warfarin dose may need to be adjusted downward.

308. ↑ warfarin (Coumadin)   **salicylates**
anisindione (Miradon)
dicumarol   aspirin
                                      Alka Seltzer, Anacin,
                                      Ascriptin, Aspergum, Bayer
                                      Bufferin, Cama, Ecotrin
                                      Empirin, Measurin
                                      Momentum, Persistin
                                      St. Joseph

Severity: ●●●
Probability: ●●●

USES: Warfarin is an anticoagulant used to thin the blood and prevent it from clotting. Aspirin is used for pain and inflammation in arthritic-type conditions and for general pain, fever, and inflammation.

EFFECT: The effect of warfarin may be increased.

RESULT: Increased risk of hemorrhage with symptoms such as bruising or bleeding anywhere on the body, black or tarry stools.

WHAT TO DO: Monitor prothrombin times and lower the warfarin dose as needed. Avoid this combination if feasible.

309. ↑ warfarin (Coumadin)   **sulfamethoxazole/
                                           trimethoprim**
                                      Bactrim, Cotrin
                                      Septra, Sulfatrim

Severity: ●●●
Probability: ●●●

USES: Warfarin is an anticoagulant used to thin the blood and prevent it from clotting. Sulfamethoxazole/trimethoprim is an antibiotic combination used for microbial infections.

EFFECT: The effect of warfarin may be increased.

RESULT: Increased risk of hemorrhage with symptoms such as bruising or bleeding anywhere on the body, black or tarry stools.

WHAT TO DO: Monitor prothrombin times and lower the warfarin dose as needed.

310. ↑ **warfarin (Coumadin)**   **sulfinpyrazone (Anturane)**

Severity: ●●●
Probability: ●●●

USES: Warfarin is an anticoagulant used to thin the blood and prevent it from clotting. Sulfinpyrazone is used for the hyperuricemia (excess uric acid in the blood) associated with gouty arthritis.

EFFECT: The effect of warfarin may be increased.

RESULT: Increased risk of hemorrhage with symptoms such as bruising or bleeding anywhere on the body, black or tarry stools.

WHAT TO DO: Monitor prothrombin times and lower the warfarin dose as needed.

311. **warfarin (Coumadin)**   **thioamines**
     anisindione (Miradon)   methimazole (Tapazole)
     dicumarol   propylthiouracil (PTU)

Severity: ●●●
Probability: ●○○

USES: Warfarin is an anticoagulant used to thin the blood and prevent it from clotting. Thioamines are antithyroid agents used for hyperthyroidism.

EFFECT: The effect of warfarin may be either increased or decreased.

RESULT: If increased: risk of hemorrhage with symptoms such as bruising or bleeding anywhere on the body, black or tarry stools. If decreased: the condition treated with warfarin may not be properly controlled.

WHAT TO DO: Monitor prothrombin times and clinical signs, and adjust the warfarin dose as needed.

312. ↑ **warfarin (Coumadin)**   **thyroid**
anisindione (Miradon)   dextrothyroxine (Choloxin)
dicumarol   levothyroxine (Synthroid)
                                   liothyronine (Cytomel)
                                   liotrix (Euthroid, Thyrolar)
                                   thyroglobulin (Proloid)
                                   thyroid (Armour Thyroid)

   Severity: ●●●
Probability: ●●○

USES: Warfarin is an anticoagulant used to thin the blood and prevent it from clotting. Thyroid hormones are used for hypothyroidism and for goiters (enlargements of the thyroid gland).

EFFECT: The effect of warfarin may be increased.

RESULT: Increased risk of hemorrhage with symptoms such as bruising or bleeding anywhere on the body, black or tarry stools.

WHAT TO DO: Monitor prothrombin times and lower the warfarin dose as needed.

313. ↑ **warfarin (Coumadin)**   **vitamin E**
anisindione (Miradon)
dicumarol

   Severity: ●●●
Probability: ●○○

USES: Warfarin is an anticoagulant used to thin the blood and prevent it from clotting. Vitamin E is an important anti-oxidant needed for stability of muscle, red blood cells, and membranes, and is necessary for normal reproduction. Sources: vegetable oils, whole-grain cereals, wheat germ, green leafy vegetables, lettuce, egg yolk, margarine, legumes (peas, beans, etc.); also available in numerous vitamin supplements (read product labels).

EFFECT: The effect of warfarin may be increased.

RESULT: Increased risk of hemorrhage with symptoms such as bruising or bleeding anywhere on the body, black or tarry stools.

WHAT TO DO: Monitor prothrombin times and lower the warfarin dose as needed.

314. ↓ **warfarin (Coumadin)**   **vitamin K**
anisindione (Miradon)   phytonadione (Mephyton)
dicumarol

Severity: ●●○
Probability: ●●●

USES: Warfarin is an anticoagulant used to thin the blood and prevent it from clotting. Vitamin K is essential for the formation of prothrombin, a substance necessary for normal blood clotting. Sources: green leafy vegetables, pork liver, vegetable oils; vitamin K also is synthesized by intestinal flora.

EFFECT: The effect of warfarin may be decreased.

RESULT: The condition treated with warfarin may not be properly controlled.

WHAT TO DO: Monitor prothrombin times and clinical response, and use a higher dose of warfarin as needed. Avoid foods or supplements containing vitamin K if possible.

Appendix:
Food-Drug
Interactions

For quick reference, potential food-drug interactions are listed together here. Though some food-drug interactions are not as strongly documented as others, it is prudent to be aware of the possibility of such interactions. Drugs are listed in alphabetical order by generic name.

↓ acetaminophen

Anacin-3, Datril, Excedrin,
Liquiprin, Panadol
Percogesic, Phenaphen
St. Joseph Aspirin-free
Tempra, Tylenol, Vanquish,
etc.

foods (high in carbohydrates)

bread, crackers, dates, jelly
etc.

USES: Acetaminophen is used for pain and fever.

EFFECT: The effect of acetaminophen may be delayed or decreased.

RESULT: Pain or fever may not be properly relieved.

WHAT TO DO: Avoid or minimize servings of high carbohydrate foods.

↓ antibiotics
erythromycin
penicillin

fruit juices (acidic)

USES: Erythromycin and penicillin are antibiotics used for microbial infections.

EFFECT: The effect of the antibiotic may be decreased.

RESULT: The infection may not be properly controlled.

WHAT TO DO: Avoid ingesting this combination at the same time.

bisacodyl (Dulcolax)

foods (alkaline-producing)

almonds, brazil nuts
chestnuts, coconut
fruit/fruit juices (except
    cranberries, plums, prunes,
    rhubarb)
milk/buttermilk, molasses
vegetables (except corn,
    dried lentils)

USES: Bisacodyl is a stimulant laxative.

EFFECT: The protective coating on the tablet may be dissolved.

RESULT: Possible severe stomach irritation, cramping, vomiting.

WHAT TO DO: Avoid or minimize servings of alkaline-producing foods. (Note: though fruit juices—listed in the foods list above—may be acidic, their ultimate reactions in the body are alkaline.)

↓ digoxin (Lanoxin)   foods (high fiber)
digitalis (Digifortis)   bran cereal, cooked leafy
digitoxin (Crystodigin)   vegetables, fruits, grains
                                               prune juice, raw vegetables
                                               whole wheat foods

USES: Digoxin and the other listed preparations are used for congestive heart failure and other heart disorders.

EFFECT: The effect of digoxin may be decreased.

RESULT: The condition treated may not be properly controlled.

WHAT TO DO: Take digoxin an hour before or two hours after high fiber foods.

↑ digoxin (Lanoxin)   licorice
digitalis (Digifortis)
digitoxin (Crystodigin)

USES: Digoxin and the other listed preparations are used for congestive heart failure and other heart disorders.

EFFECT: The effect of digoxin may be increased.

RESULT: Increased risk of adverse effects.

WHAT TO DO: Avoid natural licorice—the synthetic kind is okay.

↑ griseofulvin   foods (high fat)
Fulvicin   avocados, beef, butter
Grifulvin   cake, cream, chicken salad
Grisactin   French fries
Gris-PEG   fried chicken, etc.

USES: Griseofulvin is an antifungal agent used for ringworm infections of the skin, hair, and nails and also for certain types of bacterial infections.

EFFECT: The effect of griseofulvin may be increased.

RESULT: This may be thought of as a beneficial interaction since griseofulvin is made more effective by fatty foods.

↓ high blood pressure drugs (all)   licorice

EFFECT: The effect of the high blood pressure drug may be antagonized.

RESULT: The blood pressure may not be properly controlled.

WHAT TO DO: Avoid natural licorice—the synthetic kind is okay.

↓ levodopa (Dopar, Larodopa)   foods (high in vitamin B-6 (pyridoxine))

avocados, bacon
baker's yeast, Brewer's yeast
bran products, beef kidney
beef liver, dry skim milk
kidney beans, lentils
lima beans, malted milk
molasses, navy beans, oatmeal
pork, potatoes (sweet)
salmon (fresh), soy beans
split peas, tuna, walnuts
wheat germ, yams.

USES: Levodopa is used for Parkinson's disease.

EFFECT: The effect of levodopa may be decreased.

RESULT: The condition treated may not be properly controlled.

WHAT TO DO: Avoid or minimize servings of foods high in vitamin B-6. Option: use Sinemet (levodopa/carbidopa), which interacts minimally or negligibly with vitamin B-6. (Note: many multivitamin supplements contain vitamin B-6—read product labels.)

↕ lithium   foods (salt)
Cibalith-S
Eskalith
Lithane
Lithobid

USES: Lithium is used for manic-depressive illness.

EFFECT: A low-salt diet may increase the effect of lithium; a high salt diet may decrease the effect of lithium.

RESULT: A diet containing too little salt may cause lithium toxicity with symptoms such as dizziness, dry mouth, weakness, confusion, loss of energy, appetite loss, nausea, stomach or abdominal pain, loss of coordination. If the diet contains too much salt, the condition treated may not be properly controlled.

WHAT TO DO: Avoid a diet too low or too high in salt content. Table salt (sodium chloride) is found in a variety of foods.

↑ MAO Inhibitors

isocarboxazid (Marplan)
pargyline (Eutonyl)
phenelzine (Nardil)
tranylcypromine (Parnate)

foods (amine-containing)

avocados, baked potatoes
bananas, bean pods, beer
bologna, Brie, broad beans
caviar, cheeses
chicken liver, figs (canned)
meat tenderizers, nuts
soups (packet), pepperoni
herring (pickled)
raspberries, salami
sauerkraut, summer sausage
sour cream, soy sauce, wine
yeast, yogurt

USES: MAO inhibitors are used for some cases of clinical depression.

EFFECT: Possible dangerous rise in blood pressure. (This effect can occur even several weeks after the MAO inhibitor is discontinued.)

RESULT: Severe headache, fever, visual disturbances, confusion which may be followed by brain hemorrhage/stroke.

WHAT TO DO: Avoid amine-containing foods.

↓ methenamine

Hiprex
Mandelamine
Urex

foods (alkaline-producing)

almonds, brazil nuts
chestnuts, coconut
fruit/fruit juices (except
    cranberries, plums, prunes,
    rhubarb)
milk/buttermilk, molasses

vegetables (except corn,
dried lentils)

USES: Methenamine is used for urinary tract (bladder and kidney) infections.

EFFECT: The effect of methenamine may be decreased.

RESULT: The condition treated may not be properly controlled.

WHAT TO DO: Avoid or minimize servings of alkaline-producing foods. (Note: though fruit juices—listed in the foods list above—may be acidic, their ultimate reactions in the body are alkaline.)

phenytoin (Dilantin)

ethotoin (Peganone)
mephenytoin (Mesantoin)

↑ foods (monosodium glutamate)

food flavor enhancers
"Chinese food"

USES: Phenytoin and the other drugs listed are anticonvulsants used for seizure disorders such as epilepsy.

EFFECT: The effect of monosodium glutamate (MSG) may be increased.

RESULT: Possible toxic effects with symptoms such as weakness, numbness at back of the neck, heart palpitations.

WHAT TO DO: Avoid foods high in monosodium glutamate.

↑ quinidine

Cardioquin
Cin-Quin
Duraquin
Quinaglute Dura-Tabs
Quinalan
Quinidex Extentabs
Quinora

foods (alkaline-producing)

almonds, brazil nuts
chestnuts, coconut
fruit/fruit juices (except
cranberries, plums
prunes, rhubarb)
milk/buttermilk, molasses
vegetables (except corn,
dried lentils)

USES: Quinidine is used for heart beat irregularities.

EFFECT: The effect of quinidine may be increased.

RESULT: Possible toxic effects with symptoms such as heart palpitations or heart beat irregularities, dizziness, headache, ringing in the ears, visual disturbances.

WHAT TO DO: Avoid or minimize servings of alkaline-producing foods. (Note: though fruit juices—listed in the foods list above—may be acidic, their ultimate reactions in the body are alkaline.)

↑ **quinine**   **foods**
                                    (alkaline-producing)

Quine-260   almonds, brazil nuts
Quinamm   chestnuts, coconut
Quine   fruit/fruit juices
Quinite   (except cranberries, plums
                                       prunes, rhubarb)
                                    milk/buttermilk, molasses
                                    vegetables (except corn,
                                       dried lentils)

USES: Quinine is a nonprescription drug used for night-time leg cramps and also may be prescribed for marlaria.

EFFECT: The effect of quinine may be increased.

RESULT: Possible toxic effects with symptoms such as dizziness, headache, ringing in the ears, visual disturbances.

WHAT TO DO: Avoid or minimize servings of alkaline-producing foods. (Note: though fruit juices—listed in the foods list above—may be acidic, their ultimate reactions in the body are alkaline.)

↓ **tetracyclines**   **foods**
                                    (milk, dairy products)

demeclocycline
   Declomycin
doxycycline
   Doryx, Vibramycin, Vibra-tab
methacycline (Rondomycin)
minocycline (Minocin)
oxytetracycline (Terramycin)
tetracycline
   Achromycin V, Sumycin

USES: Tetracycline is an antibiotic used for microbial infections.

EFFECT: The effect of tetracycline may be decreased.

RESULT: The infection treated may not be properly controlled.

WHAT TO DO: Take tetracycline one hour before or two hours after ingesting milk or dairy products. (Exceptions: doxycycline and minocycline are not significantly affected by milk or dairy products.)

↓ **theophyllines**

aminophylline
  Somophyllin
dyphylline
  Dilor, Lufyllin
oxtriphylline
  Choledyl
theophylline
  Aerolate, Bronkodyl
  Bronkaid, Constant-T
  Elixophyllin, Marax, Mudrane
  Primatene, Quibron, Respbid
  Slo-bid, Slo-Phylline
  T-PHYL, Tedral, Theo-24
  Theo-Dur, Theo-Organidin
  Theobid, Theolair
  Theospan-SR, Theostat 80
  Uniphyl

foods

beef/hamburger (charcoal-
  broiled)

USES: Theophyllines are used for asthma and for bronchospasm associated with chronic bronchitis and emphysema.

EFFECT: The effect of theophylline may be decreased.

RESULT: The condition treated may not be properly controlled.

WHAT TO DO: Avoid or mimimize servings of charcoal-broiled beef or hamburger.

↓ **thyroid**

dextrothyroxine (Choloxin)
levothyroxine (Synthroid)
liothyronine (Cytomel)
liotrix (Euthroid, Thyrolar)
thyroglobulin (Proloid)
thyroid (Armour thyroid)

**foods (leafy green
  vegetables)**

asparagus, broccoli
Brussels sprouts, cabbage
kale, lettuce, peas
spinach, turnip greens
watercress

USES: Thyroid hormones are used for hypothyroidism and for goiters (enlargements of the thyroid gland).

EFFECT: The effect of thyroid may be antagonized.

RESULT: The condition treated may not be properly controlled.

WHAT TO DO: Minimize servings of leafy green vegetables.

↓ **warfarin (Coumadin)**   **foods
                                    (high in vitamin-K)**

anisindione (Miradon)   pork liver, leafy vegetables
dicumarol   (asparagus, broccoli
                                   Brussels sprouts, cabbage
                                   kale, lettuce, peas
                                   spinach, turnip greens
                                   watercress), vegetable oils

USES: Warfarin is an anticoagulant used to thin the blood and prevent it from clotting.

EFFECT: The effect of warfarin may be decreased.

RESULT: The condition treated may not be properly controlled.

WHAT TO DO: Avoid or minimize servings of vitamin-K rich foods.

Index

Please note: The numbers given are the interaction numbers, not page numbers. Also, many listings give a cross-reference. If you look up aspirin, for example, you will find:

aspirin (e.g., Anacin, Bayer) (see salicylates)

Look under *salicylates* (the "family name" for aspirin) to find listed all of the drugs that interact with aspirin.

Index of Drug Interactions

Please note: The numbers given are the interaction numbers, not page numbers.